Adam's Fall

Traumatic Brain Injury—The First 365 Days

Adam's Fall

Traumatic Brain Injury—The First 365 Days

Robert V. Bullough, Jr

SUNSTONE
PRESS

SANTA FE

Sunstone books may be purchased for educational, business, or sales promotional use.
For information please write: Special Markets Department, Sunstone Press,
P.O. Box 2321, Santa Fe, New Mexico 87504-2321.

Book and Cover design ▷ Vicki Ahl
Body typeface ▷ Constantia
Printed on acid free paper

Library of Congress Cataloging-in-Publication Data

Bullough, Robert V., 1949-
Adam's fall : traumatic brain injury-the first 365 days / by Robert V. Bullough, Jr.
p. cm.
Includes bibliographical references.
ISBN 978-0-86534-809-7 (softcover : alk. paper)
1. Bullough, Adam--Health. 2. Brain--Wounds and injuries--Surgery. 3. Head--
Wounds and injuries--Patients--Biography. 4. Brain damage--Patients--Rehabilita-
tion--Biography. I. Title.
RD594.B85 2011
617.4'81044092--dc22
[B]

2011009582

Published in

WWW.SUNSTONEPRESS.COM
SUNSTONE PRESS / POST OFFICE BOX 2321 / SANTA FE, NM 87504-2321 /USA
(505) 988-4418 / ORDERS ONLY (800) 243-5644 / FAX (505) 988-1025

Dedication

For the remarkable men and women of the SICU of Mission Hospital

Contents

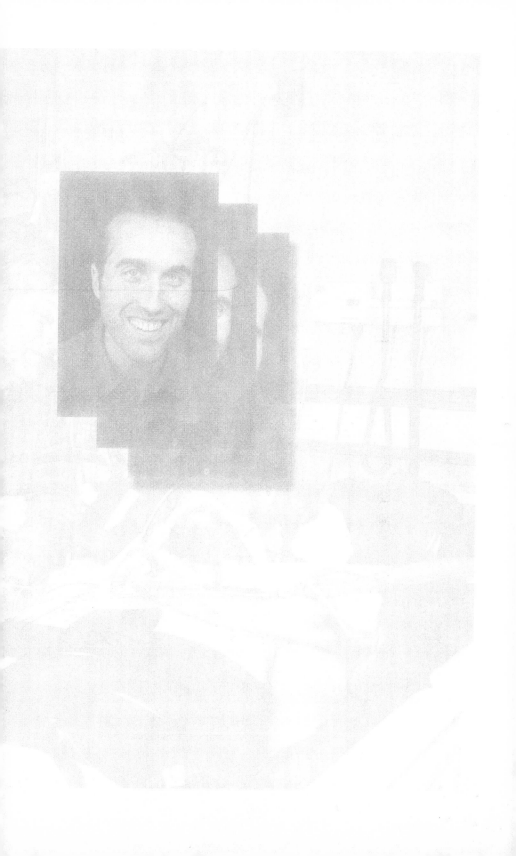

Foreword

To be honest, I entered late in this story and played only a minor role in what the reader will find a remarkable tale. That said, I have experienced the privilege of guiding a few families through similar journeys and I have attempted to help many other families when the outcomes have not been as favorable as in this story. Though I have never personally experienced the agony of watching one of my own children endure serious injury or life-threatening illness, I have often struggled with how best to help these families. I am generally an optimistic person, a person of some faith, in fact. However, is this the best attitude to adopt when dealing with patients and their families after this type of injury? I freely admit it is not always clear to me what influences the ultimate outcome of patients with severe brain trauma.

This account describes a year of roller-coaster emotions, dashed dreams and ultimately the bright hope of the Bullough family. Admittedly, reading about Adam's experience was an excruciating experience for me because he suffered most of my worst patient-care nightmares. Neurosurgeons live by the "Monro-Kellie doctrine," which states that within the fixed space of the skull there is only room for brain tissue, blood within blood vessels, and cerebrospinal fluid. Brain trauma causes swelling of the brain, which results in brain injury caused by the limited amount of space in the skull. Adam's doctors had to manipulate his physiology to prevent the damage that could be caused by this swelling. He had a tube placed in his brain to divert his cerebrospinal fluid while measuring the pressures in his brain—termed intracranial pressure. When these measures proved insufficient he required the temporary (months-long—which, in Neurosurgical parlance, is a short period of time) removal of a portion of his skull to allow space for the swollen, inflamed brain tissue. His severe head injury further required the desperate measure of purposely cooling his body temperature below normal in an attempt to protect his brain from ongoing injury caused by brain swelling.

As if this wasn't bad enough, as the intracranial pressures and brain swelling became more manageable, the focus of Adam's caregivers (and subsequently his family) shifted to his pulmonary function. Adam's decreased level of consciousness necessitated his placement on a mechanical ventilator. Lung infection—termed pneumonia—is an almost expected outcome of long-term use of the ventilator. The dreaded complication of lung injury in the mechanical ventilator-dependent patient is ARDS—Adult Respiratory Distress Syndrome. ARDS has many synonyms but the outcome is similar— many patients simply can't exchange oxygen from the lungs into the blood stream and they die when their organs starve for oxygen. As with his brain swelling, when Adam suffered ARDS, extraordinary measures were required to improve his lung function, including the placement of a tracheostomy (surgical procedure to make a direct opening into the patients breathing tube and lungs), prolonged and complicated manipulations of his ventilator and oxygen levels, placement in his bed in the prone position, and the controversial use of nitric oxide.

Through nothing short of a miracle, Adam was eventually able to be weaned from the ventilator; he had his tracheostomy, numerous intravenous lines, and gastric feeding tube removed. This is where the real struggle begins— the long and arduous journey of recovery. The reader gains an inside look at the frustration that Adam and his family experienced as he relearned how to walk, speak, read, play the guitar (most important to him) and, eventually, drive. The struggles of sorting out the financial implications of a prolonged, serious illness with hospitalization requiring complex medical procedures will be all too familiar to others that have gone through this experience.

Even with aggressive treatment, a traumatic brain injury can change an individual's personality considerably. I am often amazed at how a seemingly insignificant concussion can render a previously intelligent person incapable of multitasking, concentration, and functioning at their pre-injury level. Fortunately, with time, most of these repercussions disappear and the person returns to normal. With severe brain injury this is not always the case, but, especially in the young, it is a possible outcome. The unfortunate reality is that recovery takes time—not days or weeks, but certainly months and even years.

This book allows the medical practitioner, patient, friend, and family member dealing with severe head injury to experience the deeply personal and emotional struggle of Adam Bullough and his family through the eyes of his father Robert Bullough. This account has been stripped of all pretense. It is inspiring to read and describes not only the faith, prayers, and hope of this family but also their frustrations, doubts, and concerns for the future. This book will help physicians and nurses, as well as respiratory, physical, and occupational therapists to understand the struggles of their patients and their families. This book will bolster the faith of the family in the midst of dealing with a loved one with severe head injury. Finally, it is possible that someone currently recovering from traumatic brain injury might find comfort and hope for their recovery within the pages of this book.

—Randy Jensen, MD, PhD
Professor of Neurosurgery, Radiation Oncology,
and Oncological Sciences,
University of Utah

Preface

Traumatic brain injury. TBI. When the son of a neighbor was struck by a car while riding his bicycle and sustained a serious head injury, I recall asking questions about the nature and the extent of the injury. Until that time I hadn't thought much about injuries to the brain. Who does? Our friend's son recovered and an insurance settlement followed. Subsequently, this same young man took a tumble. Another head injury. This time the results were less favorable, and he changed, dramatically. He was no longer the person we knew. Often, when urging my own children to wear their helmets when biking, I invoked this young man's name as a reminder and a warning of what can happen.

After a long day, my wife, Dawn Ann, and I had just crawled into bed on Tuesday, August 12, when the phone rang. Dawn Ann answered. Immediately she knew something was wrong. Kirby, our son Adam's girlfriend who he was visiting in California, tearfully began speaking. She was phoning from Mission Hospital. Adam had fallen while they were riding their bikes, she said, and he was badly hurt. Somehow he had gone over the handle bars, landed on the pavement, bounced, hitting the back of his head, hard. He was then in surgery. The extent of his injuries was uncertain but they were serious. He was not wearing a helmet. We phoned our other children to tell them what had happened. Joshua and his wife Vorn, Seth, and Rachel, who was living at home, joined us for a family prayer on Adam's behalf. Additional phone calls followed; and we were told that it would be wise for us to get to California as quickly as possible. No flights were available from Salt Lake to Orange County until morning. At 1 a.m. Dr. Massoudi, a neurosurgeon, phoned from the hospital to tell us that Adam was in critical condition with a traumatic brain injury and that the surgery had gone well. Dr. Chang also phoned asking permission to conduct a bronchoscopy. Adam had aspirated vomit. Unable to sleep, at 4 a.m. we began packing to leave not knowing how long we would be away from home or what we would find once we arrived at Mission Hospital. Before departing for the airport we phoned our parents to tell them what had happened. Just a month earlier Dawn Ann's mother had died suddenly, and we did not want to add to her father's burdens. We arrived at Long Beach Airport at 9:20 a.m. where we were met by Kirby's mother, Heidi, and a family friend, Jay Mortensen, who drove as quickly as he dared to the hospital. Mostly no one spoke.

There are many causes of traumatic brain injury and symptoms vary from mild to severe depending on the extent of the injury. Our son's injuries were very severe. His fall crushed much of the back of his head. Each year in the United States 1.4 million people sustain a TBI. Of these, 235,000 are hospitalized and 50,000 die. Most traumatic brain injuries result from falls (28%), followed by motor vehicle crashes (20%). Assaults account for 11% of TBIs. Young men, like Adam, age 24, account for most serious brain injuries. TBI is a major issue for active duty service men and women in war zones. Estimates are that about 2% of the U.S. population, at least 5.3 million people, require long-term assistance with daily living because of TBI. The direct and indirect costs of TBI are staggering, running into the tens of billions of dollars. Some policies make matters worse: A few years ago the legislature of our state, Utah, repealed a law requiring motorcycle helmets as an infringement on individual rights—and many millions of dollars in medical bills and much unnecessary heartache have followed.

Adam's Fall: Traumatic Brain Injury)—the First 365 Days is written for family and friends of survivors of TBI, medical personnel, including those who care for them but also those who educate caregivers, and therapists. It may seem presumptuous to claim to have written something of value to medical personnel. This belief is based on numerous conversations with physicians, nurses and respiratory, occupational, speech, and physical therapists. For those physicians, nurses, and therapists battling TBI, the work is physically, intellectually, and emotionally exhausting; there is nothing quite like it. There are remarkable highs and devastating lows, when, despite having done all that can be done for a patient, something still goes wrong and the outcome is terrible—a life worse than death. Time and again we have been told that one of the key variables in the successful treatment of TBI is existence of an extensive and strong network of supportive and determined family and friends. Treatment is most effective when medical personnel—physicians, nurses, therapists—collaborate fully and engage the patient's family completely. To this end, knowledge of the family side of the treatment equation is indispensable. For family and friends of TBI sufferers, knowing something about the treatments being given to their loved ones is helpful as is knowledge of the range of issues that quickly follow injury, issues that can and often do prove overwhelming. Family and friends need to know that they can and should play a central role in the treatment given, that they should not hesitate to ask lots of questions, and that there is help available to them even during the darkest of days. For each of these three audiences, there is another reason for writing, perhaps an even more significant reason: to share a message of hope.

Hope is a mixed emotion. Often confused with optimism, hope is composed of a cluster of competing sentiments—dread and fear on one side, confidence and trust on the other. Unlike optimism, which brings with it an expectation of a best outcome, at least as commonly understood, hope may be present even in the most dire of circumstances and despite recognized limits to one's ability to alter and improve a situation. At such times, to maintain hope we may look outside ourselves for comfort and to cope. As such, hope serves as a basis for remaining actively engaged in life and not merely positive about it. Indeed, hope keeps us engaged and working when the smart money says give up; and, when we simply must let go and give up or in, hope often returns but in a slightly different and more mature form—flowing out of a deepening sensitivity to the full range of human experience it comes as a determination to find something good and positive in what otherwise is dreadful, an affirmation of the worth of life and the value of living despite life's challenges. There is a profound realism about hope that is lacking in optimism for hope acknowledges the very real possibility of failure. Because hoping takes us beyond our normal abilities, favorable, although often unexpected outcomes, may follow. To receive them is to live in a state of grace for a time, of having been given an undeserved gift, a miracle. Hope directs our attention simultaneously inward and outward, toward our own vulnerability and dependence and toward the well-being of those who matter most to us, those whose lives are inextricably intertwined with our own and who give our lives meaning and purpose. Hence, to give up hope *is* to give up, and what is given up is something profoundly beautiful, our very humanity.

Although tied to temperament, hope is both taught and learned. And individual hopefulness is embedded—for good or ill—in the hopefulness of others. Human networks of hopefulness or despair form and, having formed, tend to grow. Thus, some families and some cultures, including the cultures that form at work, like some individuals, are more hopeful than others and these cultures encourage individual resilience, the ability to bounce back from failure. By their very nature those who work successfully within high stress and emotionally demanding occupations like those of the Surgical Intensive Care Unit (SICU) at Mission Hospital are hopeful people. Yet, even they need help to maintain hope. Within high stress occupations a key to maintaining hopefulness is achieving valued outcomes, trust in others, consistent investment in learning and development, and recognition for and celebration of work well-done. To this end, the end of celebration, this book is dedicated to the men and women of the SICU at Mission Hospital as a token of our love, gratitude, and deep respect.

A word about reading *Adam's Fall: Traumatic Brain Injury—the First 365 Days*: This is a profoundly personal book, perhaps a bit too personal in a few places. Believing that others might benefit from his experience, Adam wants his story told. In times of deep crisis we find out who we are and what we most value. Adam has proven himself resilient and, I believe, courageous even as at times he has battled deep discouragement. We are proud of him.

To understand some parts of the story a little background information is needed, particularly information about our family. Otherwise here and there some of what is written will make no sense at all. Our faith and its supporting rituals gives form and substance to our lives. We are members of the Church of Jesus Christ of Latter-day Saints and believe in the efficacy of fasting and prayer as means for finding meaning and for coping with life's challenges. Each of our three sons have served two year "missions." Adam met Kirby and her family while on his mission in Southern California where he served and came to deeply love the Spanish language, and Latin cultures and peoples. At the time of Adam's injury I was serving as a lay minister, a bishop, which involved Dawn Ann and me intimately in the lives of about 280 single young people ages 18 to 31. For ten years Dawn Ann has been an elementary school teacher. The spring prior to Adam's tumble she had applied for and been given a new job, school librarian. In her absence, two substitute librarians kindly assumed her duties. I am employed by Brigham Young University and work in the Center for the Improvement of Teacher Education and Schooling. We live in downtown Salt Lake City but I work in Provo, Utah, 45 miles to the south. Prior to his injury Adam taught P.E. on Mondays and Wednesday's at his mother's school, worked at the Children's Museum building displays, and took classes at the community college.

The organization of *Adam's Fall: Traumatic Brain Injury—the First 365 Days* is unusual and as such may place a few unexpected demands on readers when tracking the story line. There are no chapters per se, although there are sections with thematic headings. Rather than assume a traditional narrative structure, the story primarily takes the form of an epistolary. Since before our children were born I have written letters to them detailing an assortment of life's events. When Adam was injured I continued to write finding solace in writing. These letters, entries in my personal journal written after Adam's fall and during his treatment, comprise the bulk of the book which might be visualized as a May pole with three interwoven streamers. The pole is composed of parts of letters from my journal which are introduced with a date and the words, "Dear Adam." The streamers fill out the narrative. The first streamer is made up of entries written on CaringBridge, a web site provided by Mission Hospital that enables family and friends of critically ill patients to receive daily updates that can be accessed easily by computer. Caringbridge entries appear throughout the text and are introduced in this way: "Dear Family and Friends." The second streamer is composed of brief entries from letters written to our children throughout the years and prior to Adam's accident. These are included because they provide a sense of Adam separate from the injury and recovery narrative. They are indented, italicized, and introduced in this way: "*Memory: ...*" Finally, a few *Medical Memos* are included, also indented and italicized. The *Medical Memos* are drawn from a variety of sources—references are included—and provide information that some readers will find useful for making sense of what, medically, was either being done to and for Adam or taking place within his body. Over the past several months we've learned a great deal about brain injuries and their treatment. Lastly, I should mention that many of the names included in the narrative have been changed as seemed prudent and proper.

A word of appreciation: numerous individuals have kindly read and given suggestions for improving *Adam's Fall*. In this task, Dawn Ann's guidance has been especially helpful. Special thanks go to Dr. William Chang, Dr. R. Vern Bullough, Sr., Dr. James Ballard, Ms. Jeanette Koski, Ms. Michelle Chapman, Ms. Rachel Bullough Easton, Dr. Steven Baugh, Ms. Margie Whitaker, Dr. James Jacobs and, of course, to Adam for whom reading the book proved both revealing and sometimes profoundly troubling. He's an amazing young man. Also, I must mention that our family is forever indebted to Heidi Tanaka and her daughters, Kirby and Emmely, who graciously took care of us, even allowing us to live with them during our months in California. Lastly, I am deeply grateful to Dr. Randy Jensen and to Mary Kay Bader, authors of the Foreword and Afterword.

The narrative begins the day after Dawn Ann and I flew into Long Beach Airport and continues for 365 days.

Adam's Fall

Thursday, August 14, 3:25 p.m., California time. Day 2.

Dear Adam:

A woman named Lisa Foto sat with us (Heidi, Kirby, Dawn Ann and me) while we ate sandwiches Heidi brought from home. Lisa had an aneurysm, and survived. As she shared some parts of her story I felt a heaviness come over me, realizing more and more the challenges that lie ahead of us. Her words are hopeful, however.

I just returned from visiting with you and was told that your brain is swelling and your head is not draining as it should and that they are giving you some sort of drug that will take you deeper into coma. We met the surgeon, Dr. Massoudi, who said there is "hope," and at this point we hold on to such statements.

Lots of folks have been calling and some emailing asking about you. Word of your accident is spreading quickly.

You are loved, Bud. As I look at your battered body, I feel a rush of emotion, gratitude you are alive, fear that you will not be able to overcome the challenges you now are facing, a longing for you to squeeze my hand back as I hold yours.

Last night Dr. Chang came by. Lousy bedside manner. Speaking as though reading a list, he rattled off lots of matter-of-fact details, including a devastating statement that yours is the worst "head injury" he'd ever seen— he's a pulmonary person, as Kirby points out, so maybe he doesn't know all things. I was so grateful to have your surgeon speak to us his few words of encouragement. You are in many, many people's prayers—Saturday and Sunday many will join us in a fast.

Seth just called for an update.

When talking with the nurses they said that you are young, healthy, and don't smoke are much in your favor for recovery. In addition, we think your stubbornness—or better put, your determination—may well prove to be a huge blessing.

> *Memory (age five, October): "Camping behind Molly's castle near Goblin Valley. You insisted on rock climbing with your brothers and ended up getting yourself in a spot that scared your mother to death. You were on a ledge and, rather than let Joshua help you, you kept moving further away from him, closer and closer to oblivion. Thankfully, Joshua got you and helped you get down."*

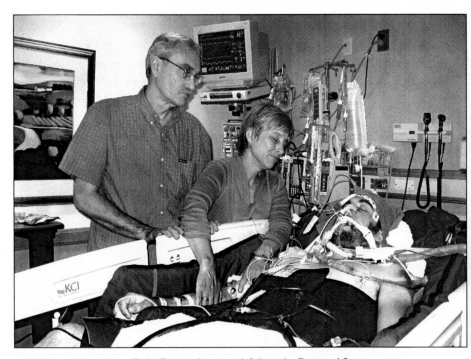

Bob, Dawn Ann, and Adam in Room 16

Dear Adam:

You have made it through another night. Today the medical people will insert a filter, described as "bird-nest" like by the nurse, into your groin area to help prevent blood clots. It turns out that after the nurses consulted with one another a decision was made to not induce a deeper coma. Other measures were taken that have helped your head drain better, the key, of course, is to reduce swelling. In part the importance of the medical people consulting one another is that the hypothermia treatment you are receiving is quite new, in fact you are one of the first in this hospital to receive it. So, there is much to learn.

This morning getting up from bed was even harder than it was yesterday. Sleep is a welcomed break from worry, even as we don't sleep all that well. Yesterday, at 6:30 I got to help turn you as the nurse, Beverly, cleaned and bandaged your wounds on your right side. It was wonderful to actually be able to do something useful.

Yesterday morning I had a conversation with the insurance people—so grateful to have insurance. While talking to Lisa, she mentioned that her final bill was $2.5 million. This figure is only now starting to sink into my head, and I worry. Somehow Lisa and her husband got on MediCal, and they are now making payments on their bill, which was mercifully reduced dramatically. I don't know what all this means for us. We don't know much about our insurance policy.

> *Medical memo: "We have found that long-term mild hypothermia significantly improves the outcome of severe TBI patients with cerebral contusion and intracranial hypertension without significant complications compared with short-term mild hypothermia. Our clinical data strongly suggest that 5 days of cooling is more efficacious than 2 days of cooling when mild hypothermia is used to control refractory intracranial hypertension in patients with severe TBI"* [1]

August 16, 1:18 p.m., California time.

Dear Adam:

The mood is a bit lighter today. You are in what the nurses describe as the "zone," meaning that the scores on the various indicators of how your body is doing are within an acceptable range. The past couple of days there has been some concern about head drainage, but today the nurse reports that the drain is working well. Apparently what happened is that a leak formed that has now sealed. This, I was told, is a common problem. A couple of hours ago the process of warming you up began which will not be complete until sometime in the early morning on August 20th. It is a very, very, gradual warming that takes place. We were told yesterday that next week, if everything goes well, you will have a feeding tube inserted into your stomach. Additionally, to lower the possibility of pneumonia, you will have a tracheotomy when you are strong enough. This is a preventative measure like having the filter placed in your groin yesterday. Each time a procedure is undertaken, it takes a while for you to bounce back.

The knuckles on your right hand look especially painful, but you can't feel anything—morphine and sedatives take care of this. All four knuckles are hard, dark red, smooth, not really knuckles at all. No broken bones other than your skull.

Mom, Emmely and Kirby added pictures to the wall surrounding your bed. The nurses are getting to know you and occasionally ask questions about the family. They seem very interested.

> *Memory (age 16, December): "Adam continues to find meaning in life in BMX bike magazines and bicycles. I don't know what that meaning is; it is encoded in a foreign tongue ('crooked pedal grinds on rails'; 'turn bar circa'; '360-one-handed x-up') and spoken to music of mumbling and screaming illiterates on video tapes that are played over and over and over again. I am certain Adam will qualify for university language credit towards a BA degree."*

It is 2 o'clock California time. August 17.

Dear Adam:

We went to church this morning, dropped by the house for a moment to change, and headed to the hospital. On the way to the hospital your mother received a phone call asking if they had permission to take you into surgery to do a craniectomy, to remove part of your skull to relieve pressure. Last night we left the hospital about 9 p.m. The nurses had been struggling to get the pressure down, but apparently over the night the situation deteriorated. On the scale they use under 20 is satisfactory, you were over 40, we were told. Dr. Massoudi, your surgeon, came in a few minutes ago and said everything went well, that they got to you "in time." The pressure has dropped precipitously, to around a 10. As we waited for word of how everything went, dark and worrisome thoughts tore at me, of having to write a final entry on your Caringbridge page and an obituary. I phoned my parents right after I spoke with your surgeon. This is very hard on them, on us all.

Naively, your mother and I thought we would be able to return home for a quick planning visit today or tomorrow. Clearly, this now not possible.

Hail Mary!

It is now 4:36 p.m. California time.

Dear Adam:

We finally got to see you. You are face down on your bed, a position that helps your lungs drain. While standing by you the nurse touched a button and the bed rapidly vibrated your body to help your lungs clear. We were told that tonight about 8 p.m. you will be turned around, face up. The surgery has lowered your brain pressure and you seem to be doing well, all things considered. When we were told that the piece of your skull that was removed will be frozen then replaced sometime between three and six months from now my heart sank. As I said earlier, I am just beginning to understand what we are up against. Your mother and I don't quite know what to do. One of us needs to get home, and soon, to meet and plan and to take care of things around the house. Silly things come to mind. The lawn mower is broken. Who knows what the lawn looks like? Lots to do. Yet, nothing matters but you and our family.

Monday, August 18. 12:52 p.m. California time.

Dear Adam:

We arrived today at the hospital but were not allowed to see you. You had a very difficult night and the oxygen levels in your brain have deteriorated. In his list-reading and affectively flat way Dr. Chang said you have "deteroriated since Friday." Not helpful, but apparently truthful and not easy to say. About 30 minutes ago Christine, one of the nurses, came out to where Kirby, your mother and I were sitting outside—we had just said a prayer—and told us they were about to turn you again on your stomach and that if we wanted we could come see you. Of course we did. You have been turned once again on your stomach which helps your lungs drain and helps you breath—it looks incredibly miserable. You are breathing 100 percent oxygen. This morning your brain/oxygen level number hovered around 15, 20 is acceptable. We swing between extreme emotions at every dip or rise in the numbers. I fixate on them. Everyone is exhausted.

August 18.

Dear Family and Friends,

The reality that under the best of conditions Adam is in for a very long period of rehab is beginning to settle in. Dawn Ann and I are not yet certain when either one of us can leave for a visit home. This must wait until we are more certain about the future—imagine that, hoping for some certainty about the future.

August 19.

Dear Adam:

It was a week ago tonight that this nightmare began. Yesterday and today have been very difficult. It is now 6:55 p.m. California time and the nurse's shift change is about to take place. Mom, Kirby and Heidi are still in with you saying "good night."

It's been another very rough day. About 35 minutes ago Mom and I visited you. Christine said that they threw a "hail Mary" and you caught it. They tried an experimental and somewhat controversial procedure with you using nitric oxide gas which is usually used only on premature infants. In some patients, it causes pulmonary vasodilation which means that blood flow improves so oxygen levels increase but not indiscriminately. It dilates blood vessels in those parts of the lung that are actively involved in gas exchange. Your lungs are damaged from having aspirated vomit when you fell and from breathing so much pure oxygen. Your blood oxygen levels were really bad for much of the day. By our second, "good night" visit, the numbers jumped. As Dave, your respiratory therapist said, you are a "responder." Christine looked at us, smiled, and gave a "thumbs up." "I love this," she said, quietly. I immediately felt relief flow over me. They've been turning you, vibrating you and moving you from side to side all to help your lungs. The book on traumatic brain injury we were given when we arrived at Mission Hospital warns that lung problems typically follow at 5 to 7 days, yours hit at 6. Aspirated vomit. I have asked when we might expect your lungs to clear and was told there is no way of knowing.

Medical memo: "What we currently know of the effects of [nitric oxide] in adults can be easily summarized. Inhaled NO is a selective pulmonary vasodilator; minute doses administered to patients with pulmonary hypertension and/or hypoxemia can rapidly decrease pulmonary artery pressure and improve the PaO2, without obvious systemic effects or toxicity. These potential benefits have been consistently reported in patients with acute respiratory distress syndrome (ARDS)..." [2]

"On the basis of the evidence, inhaled nitric oxide is not an effective intervention in patients with acute lung injury or ARDS, and its underlined routine (underlining inserted) use to achieve this end is inappropriate." [3]

7:28 p.m. California time. Day 8, August 20.

Dear Adam:

Kirby and I said "goodnight" to you just before 7 p.m. as the shift was about to change. You've had a good day. You are battling pneumonia but this is an anticipated complication, and you were started on antibiotics early. These either have been or will soon be targeted to the specific bug you've developed. You continue to be shaken and rolled and have your lungs periodically cleaned—part of a bronchoscopy. Your numbers have been much better and right now you are on 65 percent oxygen, which is a great improvement. There is a much lighter feeling in the intensive care unit among those working with you. Tonight you will have only one nurse. Today you had two.

Today I booked a flight for Rachel who will arrive tomorrow at 10:30 a.m. at the John Wayne Airport. When I last spoke with her she was purchasing stuff she needs for the stay here. I'll be very glad to see her. On the way from the airport tomorrow we will have to do a little preparation so that seeing you won't be too much of a shock for her. You are very swollen, in fact your hands look blue, as though they are on the verge of exploding from the finger tips. Your eyes are swollen shut and your head is huge, inflated.

> *Memory (age 16, August): "Rachel and Adam went fishing on the Weber River with Grandpa Bullough on Thursday, and both caught one fish. Dad caught several but didn't take any home... When Rachel got home from fishing she was proud to report that she gutted and scaled each fish and cut off their heads. 'It's fun,' she said. She reported that last time they went fishing she thought this sort of thing was disgusting, but it doesn't bother her any more. I asked Adam why she started to do this and he said, 'Because I taught her how and she is a horrific kid'."*

6:30 p.m. California time, August 21.

Dear Adam:

On the whole you have had a good day, mostly stable. One of the drain tubes was removed from your head, which is a good sign. Each tube presents an opportunity for infection, so any removal is a plus. The nitric oxide treatment continues and apparently remains effective. The antibiotics have not yet kicked in. Your lungs remain a serious concern. Your mother was told today that your CAT scans haven't changed, and that there are four places "of concern." These include parts of the brain associated with comprehension, memory, balance, and language. We are unclear just what this means. During lunch today one of the nurses, Beverly, sat with us for a while. She's very interested in you. In fact, she hopes she will be assigned to work with you on her next shift. I tried to get her to say a bit about what these spots might mean but she was wisely circumspect, noting, as is common, that each person is very different and it is hard to say. We discussed how the brain is always losing cells as it ages, that it doesn't generate new cells and, of course, that there is all sorts of potential redundancy built in such that if one part is injured another part may adapt and pick up the damaged function.

Rachel flew in today from Salt Lake City, arriving at 10:30. On the way to the hospital your mother and Heidi prepared her for what she would see. When she arrived she was exhausted, having not slept much since your accident, and wound tightly with concern and worry. As I write, Rachel has lightened up and is happily chatting with your mother. I'm grateful for this.

Heidi told your mother that last night Kirby had a "melt down." She continues to worry about what will happen when you wake up—"Will he remember me?"

Rachel told me that before you fell she had a dream of entering a room filled with toys, wooden puppets and tin wind-up toys, and "stuff like that." In the middle was a baby boy, dressed in yellow and in a wooden square crib, that she knew was one of the "boys" in our family. She didn't know if the baby was you or Seth. She picked it up and knew that she must care for and protect him. She couldn't stop thinking about the dream, worrying about it. She actually told Mom about the dream before you got hurt. Now, she is here.

ARDS

Friday, August 22, 4:50 p.m. California time.

Dear Adam:

I just came in from visiting you. Once again you are face down, so the turning, shaking, and rolling, continues. Sometime in the next little while, perhaps an hour, you are scheduled to have your lungs drained. This is done by inserting a needle into your side and into your lung and sucking the fluid out. When we asked earlier this afternoon about whether or not the antibiotics have kicked in, we were told that you are still receiving a range of drugs. You are still breathing nitric oxide—and 80 percent pure oxygen.

I neglected to mention something we were told yesterday, I believe it was by Linda, your nurse who was on duty the night you were taken to the hospital. Apparently when you first arrived you were able to answer questions— "What is your name?", "Where do you live?" We had no idea that you were still conscious. We were told that this was a very good sign. You "crashed" shortly after being admitted.

Rachel seems to be settling in. She, Kirby and Emmely talked until fairly late last night. Heidi and the girls have set up an inflatable mattress for her in the room where you stayed. She and Kirby just got back from walking to the bank together. They seem to like one another a lot.

Medical memo: "The acute respiratory distress syndrome (ARDS) is characterized by inflammatory lung injury with alveolar flooding and abnormalities in surfactant function... The syndrome is both common (with an incidence of about 80 cases per 100,000 population every year) and lethal (with a death rate of more than 38 percent) in a community population of patients with acute lung injury." [4]

"Overall, prone positioning helps to improve gas exchange in approximately two thirds of patients with ARDS... [With the] established safety, the frequent gas exchange improvement, and the potential beneficial effects on ventilator-induced lung injury that are associated with prone positioning, I do not see any compelling reason not to turn my next patient with severe ARDS to the prone position." [5]

4:02 California time, Saturday, August 23. Day 11.

Dear Adam:

It was a very rough morning for you. We were told that you have Acute Respiratory Distress Syndrome (ARDS), meaning that your lungs are not working well and your oxygen levels have deteriorated. Apparently you had been moved onto your stomach and you didn't respond well; you had to be turned over quickly—"He doesn't like it," we were told. We had anticipated that you would have the fluid in your lungs drained last night or early this morning, but the procedure wasn't done. Christine, your nurse, told us that you were going to have an ultrasound and the hope was that you would have a sufficient amount of accumulated fluid—localized—to justify the procedure. Happily, you did and its removal helped greatly. More than a liter of fluid was removed from your right lung alone. As I write your oxygen levels are set at 75, which is still high but better than 100 percent. They have set your breathing rate at 22, which also is high, as a way of containing the damage done to your lungs by highly concentrated oxygen and giving some room to expand if needs be. You will be given a diuretic by drip to help eliminate fluid and we were told that your body temperature might be raised as well which also will help with elimination. I asked about the white cell counts and was told they'd been fluctuating. At some point you will be given a transfusion with oxygen enriched blood.

Christine told me this morning that she thought you'd be better today than you are. We thought so too yesterday. The extreme swings continue. Waking up in the morning is difficult and each of us frets as we approach the hospital hoping and praying for some good news.

The chaplain here is Howard Young, a kind and good man. In a local newspaper he is featured conducting a funeral for a 14 year-old boy who died after being hit by a car while riding a skate board. The boy survived for four days in Mission Hospital. Very sad.

Last night just before saying "good night" Rachel, your mother and I sang to you, some of the oldies, the Drifters and Elvis—"Wise men say...".

5:03 California time, Sunday, August 24.

Dear Adam:

As like so many mornings, Mom and I were awake very early worrying. We hoped to be able to go to church today but didn't want to leave until we found out how you were doing. Church begins at 9:30. After the shift change, and with some encouragement, your mother phoned the hospital. She said she was afraid to call. So was I. "How is Adam doing?" "Do you think we could go to church this morning?" The drive to the hospital takes only about 5 minutes, but it is a very long time, heavy. Each morning we arrive hoping that good news will be forthcoming and dreading bad news. Upon arriving the doors to the Surgical Intensive Care Unit (SICU) were open and Heidi and I went straight in while your mother took her things to the waiting room. We were greeted by two smiling girls, Rachel and Kirby. Wonderful.

Christine was back on duty. She said you were doing "better." Yesterday worried her as well. Your oxygen numbers were up. The fluid draining from your head is almost clear—very little blood. You were strong enough to begin rolling again. You were being warmed and there was "marked improvement" in your lungs. Later in the day Christine said that warming you up was "huge," and that it was going beautifully, that you were tolerating the change very well. Apparently being warmed makes all sorts of procedures possible. She explained that slowly you have to be taken off of the interventions—the nitric oxide, cooling, and who knows what else? As I write you are still breathing 90 percent pure oxygen, but your breaths are short and not deep (respiration rate of 24) which is done to protect the lower lobes of your lungs allowing some healing. The goal is to get back to treating your head injury.

Hearing this was thrilling.

> *Medical memo: "Four therapeutic strategies appear to be the most promising approaches currently in clinical trials for severe traumatic brain injury: a) the novel pharmacologic agent dexanabinol; b) hypertonic saline; c) mild hypothermia; and d) decompressive craniectomy. Each of these therapies share the common feature of targeting multiple mechanisms, suggesting this may be an important factor to the development of a successful approach to severe traumatic brain injury."* [6]

5:40 p.m. California time, August 26. Day 14.

Dear Adam:

You had a very good morning and we were all in quite good spirits. Now, as I write, you have taken a turn for the worse. Your lungs continue to be a major problem and your oxygen levels dropped dramatically. Kirby, who starts classes tonight, is walking outside somewhere, doing her best to cope. Mom has been holding Rachel. Heidi has been in tears. You are on your stomach again, and they're trying to clear and strengthen your lungs. About an hour ago Dr. Chang scoped your lungs and afterwards spoke with us stating that you had a lot of damage—now, there is a surprise. He felt compelled to review with us the levels of cognitive functioning that you might have—or not have. It seemed he was preparing us to have you removed from life support. Stunned, your mother said, "We're not there yet, we are hopeful." Taken aback, he quickly responded, apparently aware of having gone too far, "No, we're not there yet."

6:47 p.m., Tuesday, August 26th, a few minutes shy of 2 weeks since your accident. I wish we knew how it was you fell off your bicycle. Probably we will never know.

Dear Adam:

Yesterday was a very rough day, one that pushed us to near despair. Your mother and I slept very little and did a lot of praying. On the way to the hospital none of us said much of anything. I'm grateful for Penny Lane, that silly dog of Heidi's. She has provided a much welcomed diversion and many light moments for the girls.

As we walk toward to the hospital from the parking lot a heaviness settles over us; I feel my body dragging. We were relieved to find that you had a pretty good night.

We were just in your room—room 16—and your numbers were also pretty good. You were face up, swollen from having spent about four hours prone and being turned from side to side.

Rachel had a long talk with your nurse, Michelle, today. They are now buds, I think. Michelle has been very encouraging. She and Daniel (who is Ukranian) are pretty funny. He's not hesitant to disagree with what others say and sometimes, as one of the respiratory therapists said, they squabble "like a married couple."

Your condition changes rapidly.

"If he were my brother, I'd…"

Dear Family and Friends,

Tomorrow we will be meeting with a medical team to decide what should be done for Adam. His strong little body is wearing down and his lungs are very sick. We will be fasting starting after lunch today for guidance about what we should do. We know that Adam would not want to live unless he could find joy in living. While we continue to hope and pray for a miracle—today another new technology was tried—what we want might not be what Adam would want or the Lord has in store for our beloved son. If you would like to join us in our fast we will be most grateful. With love, Bob and Dawn Ann.

It is 6:05 California time, Wednesday, August 27, day 15.

Dear Adam:

This is probably the last letter I will ever write to you my dear son. You are in room 16 surrounded by people who love you, Heidi, Kirby, Emmely, your Mom, Rachel, among others, including for a time Christine your nurse who has been so kind to us. You have fought a valiant fight, more than anyone could possibly ask. In the background your music is playing. Tonight Joshua, Seth…I almost wrote "Adam"…and Vorn will fly in. Tomorrow morning Aunt Patio, Aunt Tammy, Aunt Beckie and Grandpa Mortensen will come. Our hearts are broken. How I wanted you to be a daddy. How I looked forward to hearing you sing every morning when you were small, and singing then playing your guitar as you grew—you wouldn't let me hear you play but I'd sit outside your door and listen. As your music played one of the nurses came over, a male nurse, and asked whose music was playing. "His," Daniel said. He was impressed. Now, the music is slowly dying. I feel so grateful that you were my son and so sad that I wasn't a better father to you. I was too professionally ambitious and too neglectful of the important things of life. You are beloved, Adam. I still have just a spark of hope that you will return to us now, but I also know that you are very tired and that your lungs have little life left in them.

Your Mom and I love you with all our hearts and do not know how we will face living without you. But, we will in anticipation of seeing you again.

Love, Dad

Day 16. August 28.

Dear Adam:

The last letter I wrote I was broken hearted. Now...a miracle.

It is 7:35 p.m. California time. At 5:30 we met with the medical team that is caring for you. Dr. Massoudi began the meeting saying that there is lots of healthy brain tissue and while there is considerable damage, if you were his brother he would keep doing what is being done. He said there is hope. Having expected the worst, I was stunned and cried. He said that you will have difficulties particularly with speech—I said that maybe you'd confuse Spanish and English. While he spoke cautiously, I mentioned that you are a stubborn and a rather remarkable little guy who often surprises and we expect you to surprise us again. You have considerable damage primarily to the back of your head but, we were told, there is a lot of salvageable, good, brain matter left. Dr. Massoudi said there is also hope in future research, mentioning specifically stem cell research. The room was filled: Aunt Patio, Heidi, Kirby, Mom, me, Aunt Amy Sue, Ashley, your cousin Jackie's wife, Beckie, Grandpa Mortensen, Tammy, Joshua, Vorn, Seth, Rachel. Michelle, your nurse, who has cried with us—more, she said, than she has cried in the "last ten years"—was there and later Dr. Chang joined us. Dr. Chang said that he couldn't explain the improvement he's seen over the past 12 hours—we can, people all over the country have fasted and are praying for you—but it has been significant. He said he is "cautiously optimistic." You began the day, early, at 100 percent oxygen and are at 60 percent now. Your lungs, while badly damaged, are showing signs of moving through to a second phase of APD (Acute Pulmonary Distress), which apparently is good. You are not in as deep a coma as you have been and you are off the two drugs that help maintain your blood pressure—both of these are very good developments. As I write you are in the "zone".

At the end of the meeting, I asked your Grandpa Mortensen to give a prayer and I asked those present to join us if they wished. Dr. Chang, Howard Young the chaplain, and Pam Kennard, an RN, stayed (Michelle and Dr. M. were gone by then). Your Grandpa expressed gratitude for the news received and pronounced a blessing on the medical personnel taking care of you for whom we are deeply grateful.

After the meeting we went into your room and excitedly gathered around. Daniel gave me a joyful hug. I even hugged Dr. Chang, asking permission first, however. And Michelle hugged everyone.

I should mention that Daniel urged us to talk to you and to play music. He told me that many patients remember being talked to and hearing music— although they may not know what is said, they "hear" he said. Rachel brought your songs.

Adam, my faith has been sorely tested. Your mother has passed her test. The future is uncertain but I feel lighter, as though I've been given a second chance. And the music plays on!!

> Medical memo: "Upon injury, adult CNS (Central Nervous System) axons undergo a spontaneous, but short-lived and ultimately abortive attempt at repair called regenerative sprouting."[7]

> "Collateral sprouting is a common response of the CNS to injury. It was first described in the spinal cord and shortly thereafter in the brain. Since then, lesion-induced forms of neuronal plasticity

*have been demonstrated in numerous species and brain regions...
Accordingly, sprouting processes occur following head traumata
where a singular massive loss of nerve cells takes place..."* [8]

*"The plasticity of the brain and the rewiring of neural connections
make it possible for one part of the brain to take up the functions of
a disabled part."* [9]

A Strange Fellowship

Dear Adam:

Dave the respiratory therapist was really on his game today. I think he was feeling his oats a bit, having saved your life by suggesting use of nitric oxide, a procedure never used here before on an adult. He was quite aggressive today, removing you from nitric oxide precipitously rather than gradually. At first, you did very well with the change, but, as he said later, you "like" nitric oxide. You were being given 20 parts per million then 10 then none. You hit a bad patch, and he took you back to 10. Most of the day you were at 55 to 60 percent oxygen and you, as they say, "stayed in the zone." The bad patch lasted perhaps an hour.

There was some difficulty finding a vein in your right arm so that your blood could be tested. You're a pin cushion. An ultra sound was actually used to find a vein. In any case, Dave got you stable again which was a huge relief. I'm not certain I could have taken another serious downturn.

At one point during the time when your numbers had slipped (from 26 to 13-14-15 in minutes) Dave began tapping your back with his hands cupped. I asked him, "could I do that?" "Sure," he said and moved aside. When I tapped a bit too aggressively, he cupped his hands and patted me demonstrating the desired level of intensity. As I wrote on today's Caringbridge update, the temptation to pound hard and drive the crud out of your lungs was strong. Seth joined in tapping.

Here I should mention something that happened to Kirby a couple of days after your accident. She, Heidi and Emmely were watching the Olympics when Kirby fell sort of half way asleep. She had been feeling all sorts of doubts about your love for her and your relationship. She said that she looked up and you were looking over her, that she started and she called your name. She thinks you came to her to comfort her.

A dear friend, Matthew Lampros, flew in for the day. He brought with him a book about and pictures of his best friend in high school, Vince. Vince was a mountain climber and competitive athlete, smart and talented, who was injured in a biking accident—wearing a helmet, he landed on top of his head and was paralyzed from the waist down. Matthew phoned Vince and asked him about his experience. Apparently Vince's parents were told that there was no point in continuing treatment, that he was too badly damaged to recover and have a productive life. They decided otherwise—and he not only lived but got an electrical engineering degree, has a full time job, and soon will be married. He has some lingering problems and has endured a very long period of rehabilitation, but the story is quite amazing. Vince assured Matthew he was glad to be alive.

The nurses today gave your mom a present—your shorn locks. I smelled them, and despite my perpetually clogged nose, smelled you. The other day when feeling pretty low your mother and I went through some of your clothes and pulled out a couple of things you had worn and smelled them. Odd, perhaps, but comforting to both of us.

Now, a summary of the day according to Dave the respiratory therapist: "He had a great day." Perhaps, just perhaps, my dear Adam, you are turning the corner that we've so longed for.

Norbert (Adam's PacMan toad) is doing great. He doesn't have a clue that anything is going on and is still enjoying eating his "pinkies."

Saturday, August 30, 5 p.m., California time.

Dear Adam:

Today has been a relatively quiet day. For quite some time you were off the nitric oxide, but you are now on it again. Apparently your oxidation numbers dropped some as the day progressed. You were given castor oil to help your bowls get flowing. I spoke with one of the pulmonary physicians today who said that next couple of days are very important, that your lungs need to begin to show some signs of improvement—developing new tissue and not serious scarring. Developing new tissue is crucially important to your healing and future health. You continue to be turned front to back and side to side but there hasn't been any shaking. The reason for this is that you don't have any appreciable fluid in your lungs. Instead, you have fluid in the sack surrounding the lungs, which is apparently difficult to treat.

When this nightmare began we were told that people in coma liked being touched but not rubbed or petted. So, what do we do?—rub and pet. We do this because it is comforting to us, to feel your body and to express our love in ways that otherwise would seem natural. So, Adam, when you wake up, forgive us for irritating you—but then, love often has irritating effects.

You are still breathing "on your own" from time to time but I was told today that the nurses would rather you did not, that to do so takes energy. Yet somehow we find this encouraging.

I am not certain any of us here understands how long it is going to take for you to recover even as everyone undoubtedly feels deeply the uncertainty of the future.

A quiet day is a good day, but we need days that signal clear improvement. We are not used to sicknesses of the kind you have, one's that require long term, slow, painful, recoveries. We somehow expect quick recoveries, like when having a cold, and then impatience sometimes prompts us to ignore what we know we should do with the result that a cold lingers. You remain, Adam, a very sick young man.

Dear Adam:

We attended church this morning and were rather slow getting to the hospital, much to my frustration. When we arrived you were on your stomach and being rocked back and forth. Your numbers were amazing, despite looking very uncomfortable—46 on the brain oxygen levels, which is very good. When you were flipped onto your back the numbers slipped quite a lot, although they gradually rose to around 30, still good. A decision was made to put you on your stomach again and to keep you there for longer periods of time. Felipe, a respiratory therapist, was thrilled with how well you did and removed you from nitric oxide. The blood tests suggested that it wasn't helping any more, he said. Around 6 o'clock he got a bit frustrated, saying that you were "kicking his butt." Your numbers had dropped to 26, although the oxygen saturation level of your body (which is separate from the head) was very good. He and your nurse struggled to get you into a position that you liked. As we left Felipe was speaking with Rob, the therapist who will be on duty tonight, about what he had done and what he thought was going on. One of the difficulties was positioning the air tubes so they wouldn't kink. Your face was basically stuck in a pillow, your nose flattened, and as you were moved there appeared to be some difficulty with the tubes. Rob suggested cutting a pillow to better fit your face, which made a lot of sense to me. Also, you won't be rocked for a time which will allow your arms to be extended from your body. This, Felipe suggested, is a better position for you in part because nothing is coming up when your lungs are suctioned, and rocking is designed to break up mucus. You still have fluid around your lungs, which remains a concern. But, all in all today you made some progress. Most especially your lungs have opened up more, widened, which is very important to generating new and healthy tissue.

We continue to pray that you will turn a corner and begin making greater positive strides, but it is clear that this will be a very, very, slow process.

Early in the morning Grandpa Mortensen, Aunt Tammy, and Aunt Beckie leave for home. Josh, Vorn, Seth and Aunt Patio left around 3:15 today. It was difficult for them to leave and comforting to have them here but having so many people in Heidi's house for much longer would have been a bit straining, I think. Heidi, Emmely and Kirby need to return to their beds. Heidi and Kirby slept on the floor and Emmely on a couch. On Tuesday Heidi begins her pre-school again. She is looking forward to it. Getting back into some routines will be much welcomed. There is comfort in predictability.

Last night the nurse told me that it is important not to overstimulate you and accordingly your mother and I have told everyone that we need to be more sensitive when visiting. There was a bit too much laughter and goofing around by the girls yesterday even as I understand how important it is for us to smile and be happy, not so gloomy. There is much to be grateful for. Also, we've cut down on the number of people who visit at one time. Last night, late, as I was talking to and singing to you, just you and me, the nurse said that you seemed to respond positively to my touch and voice and that I should "keep it up." I was thrilled even though I know you probably cannot hear me.

August 31.

Dear Family and Friends,

A word about Genevieve, Adam's nurse for the past three days. Genevieve is a quiet and remarkably focused person who moves slowly, calmly, and deliberately. Watching her and the other nurses each of whom has his or her own way of going about their business and getting to know them has been an unexpected blessing and deepened our appreciation for who these people are and what they do. Today Genevieve asked to hear some of Adam's music. Her request was touching but not just kind. She was genuinely interested. It is amazing how everyone caring for Adam has connected to him and how deeply invested they are in his well-being.

September 1, Labor Day, the 20th day since your accident. 4:40 p.m., California time.

Dear Adam:

You have had mostly a good day. Your LICOX numbers (a scale measuring brain oxygenation) have been good except for a short time when you were removed completely from nitric oxide. Apparently, you really like the stuff. Every time you are removed from it your numbers drop. The other day Dave, the respiratory therapist, said you needed to be slowly weaned from it but since then two other therapists have tried cold turkey on you and it's failed. Right now you are on a very low level, about 1.5 parts per million. Seeing those numbers drop really upset me. Seeing them rise was thrilling. They are also working to get the ratio of your in-breathing to out-breathing more normal. I guess at one point you were 4 to 1; normal is 1 to 2 (in to out). You are now 2 to 1. I had a discussion with Steve, your nurse today, about morphine. He mentioned that you metabolize the drug very quickly, which is unusual, so you have been given higher than normal doses. When the time comes apparently methadone is used to wean patients from their addictions. Boy, so many strange things to consider—and you don't even take aspirin for a headache. Dr. Massoudi came by this morning and in his reassuring way said, smiling, "His numbers are good."

Dee, one of the women here whose husband is battling for his life—your mother wrote on Tom's Caringbridge page and today I noticed Dee had written on your page—just came over to talk with us about what is going on with her husband, that she was told to leave while they "turned him." Your mother explained what is being done and shared a few insights with her. The people here bond in various ways. There's a little boy, Jose, a Mexican, who is as cute and as bright as he can be. His brother fell out of a tree and has been in care for 9 months—mostly here. Apparently they are undocumented and have no insurance. The family makes ends meet by tree cutting—a bit of rope would have saved his brother. Another Hispanic family joined us today, a young boy, we think. So sad. There is a woman here named Karen who has friends visit each day. Today she sat up and it was cause for celebration. The food Heidi brings is often shared. Today half a chocolate cake was given to the nurses. We are part of a very strange fellowship, Adam, one that no one ever imagines joining.

Memory (age 8, November): "I asked you as you came home from school how your day had been. 'Good, except I had two headaches and almost threw up in class.' 'Oh, do you want to lie down,' I asked. 'No, I stayed in from recess and the other headache, I toughed out.' And this was a 'good' day?! Now, that's what I'd call a positive attitude."

Reversible!?

Dear Adam:

Just a few minutes ago I spoke with Dr. Chang who said he thought the ARDS has peaked and he sees signs of improvement. You have had 3 mostly good days, which is a miracle, truly a miracle. We fasted again Sunday to Monday and you are constantly in our and many other people's prayers. This morning Dave is back. He inspires feelings of confidence in me. Michelle is your nurse (who gave hugs to everyone when we walked in). The nitric oxide bottles are gone as is the paralytic. You are still on your stomach. Dave succeeded in cleaning some more stuff out of your lungs this morning, which is good.

Last night while we were in the SICU waiting room during the shift change (7 to 8 p.m.) a physician entered and spoke with Dee. Dee is a remarkable and very kind person. Tom hit a deer while riding his motorcycle and is not doing well. (I just noticed Tom's will is sitting on the desk next to me) To top it off, he has cancer and was supposed to start chemo a few days ago. Earlier today Dee spoke with us about Tom and your mother and I shared our experience with you. The physician said that Tom's organs are shutting down and the family needed to meet immediately to decide what they wanted done. As Dee cried your mother held her hand, trying to comfort her. The physician left and phone calls were made to family members and friends. Later they gathered in the same conference room where our family met last Thursday. It's a chilly room so your mother made arrangements to get blankets and I gathered up boxes of tissues. We were asked to guide folks as they entered the area—friends into the waiting room; family inside for the meeting. Tom was stable during the night, but your mother just told me that he now has ARDS, something, my dear Adam, that you know much about, know bodily, deeply. Watching your mother was amazing. I described the people here as belonging to a fellowship—we are also something of a family.

September 2.

Dear Family and Friends,

Today we received a big box of letters from the children at Wasatch Elementary School where Adam taught P.E. One of our favorites states: "How are you doing? How are you feeling? Do you get room service?" Another reads: "I was sorry to hear you were flung over your handle bars." Many said Adam was their favorite P.E. teacher. Lots mentioned that he'll be wearing a helmet for a long time since he has a big hole in his skull. We've put some of the letters on the wall of Adam's room. Thank you children and thank you Wasatch faculty for your kind and consistent support of Adam and our family.

It is 5:02 California time, still day 21—just shy of 3 weeks since your accident.

Today, my dear Adam, you have exceeded yourself.

First, some amazing news: This morning Dr. Massoudi found us in the hallway, "Oh, there you are," he said, and proceeded to give us the best news we have had since you entered the hospital—he said, smiling, that he had reviewed your CAT scan and that the damaged areas in your brain have improved even from three days ago, that the swelling is down, and that he thinks there is a very good chance that your injuries are "reversible." REVERSIBLE. HOW IS THAT!

When we arrived at the hospital today you were on your stomach and doing pretty well but now you are on your back—which you haven't liked—and your numbers are 30 and 6 and your PEEP is 10! (This has to do with the pressure in your lungs—positive end-expiratory pressure) If you hold at a 10, you will be positioned to have a trache. Your mouth looks so very sore from the tubes and infection remains a concern, so this is very important.

Now, even neater stuff: Michelle took a pen and pressed it on the top of your nail on your middle finger and, not liking it, you clinched your hands. When she pressed the pen to your big toe nail you shuddered. Who would think that a "shudder" would be thrilling?! As I mentioned in my earlier missive today, there is now good evidence that the ARDS has peaked. You still look like a fella who lost a 15 round fist fight, but we think you look great. Everyone is lighter. Dave is so pleased with himself—he and so many others have had to work very hard to get you to where you are right now, Adam, very hard—and very smart.

Wednesday, September 3, 4:31 p.m. California time. Day 22.

Dear Adam:

As I write you are in surgery. This morning we met briefly with Dr. Chang who said, and I quote, that he had viewed your latest chest x-ray and the results were "amazing." "Amazing," not "good," not "better," not "improving," not "showing signs of only modest tissue damage..." But.... Amazing! Then, he said, that for the first time he felt confident that you are "going to make it." To these words, your mother said, "We knew it Thursday." Nothing really more needed to be said. After Dr. Chang left, smiling, Rachel and Kirby did "happy feet". Then, we did a "group hug" (Mom, Kirby, Rachel and me).

According to Dave you had a "great" night. Dave allowed me to listen to your lungs through his stethoscope. All I heard, and admittedly I don't hear much, was air moving. Dave's certainly been on his game and feeling it yesterday and today. While feeling mighty good and mighty blessed, we went in to see you. Your numbers were wonderful: 34 for oxygen to the brain; 3 for head pressure; 8 for PEEP. Although assigned to another patient, Daniel, who worked his heart out for you, came in and gave us hugs. Shortly thereafter we were told that you were doing so well that it was decided to do the tracheotomy and insert the two feeding tubes, one into your small intestine and the other into your stomach. Given this news, doing phoning updates this morning was delightful.

Surgery began about 4 p.m. So, now we wait.

I cannot help but think about how we felt a week ago. Last Wednesday we were told that you were deteriorating and a decision needed to be made about your future. Then came the scrambling to get family members here, then the terrible and heavy waiting for Thursday's meeting, then the thrilling statements of both Dr. Massoudi and Dr. Chang. Now this.

Your mother and I offered a prayer of thanksgiving.

Love, Dad

Life Goes On....

Thursday, September 4, 10:30 a.m., California time. Day 23.

Dear Adam:

Yesterday your mother and I went for a walk around the area of Heidi's house. She does this every morning. As we rounded a corner, exiting the horse trail, and back onto the pavement she mentioned that we were near the place where your accident occurred. For the life of me, I cannot figure out what happened. There isn't anything obvious that could have tripped up your bicycle. I've looked the bike over pretty carefully and there isn't anything that could account, mechanically, for your being tossed. There is one broken spoke on the back wheel which is slightly warped but still turns although not cleanly—there's a slight catch with the rear brake. I'd expected problems with the front wheel, but nothing. The damage to the rear wheel likely happened when you fell. The brakes are fine and so are the tires. When you awaken perhaps you'll be able to shed some light on just what happened.

Today Kirby went back to work at the school with Emmely. Kirby was hestitant to return to work, but we urged her to. She needs to get back into her life even as we all continue to focus on you and your well-being.

The Tracheotomy surgery went well.

Your liver is swollen which complicated implanting the two feeding tubes. You have a large bandage on your stomach covering what is essentially an open wound. Once the swelling in your liver abates, the wound will be closed. I was confused about the function of the tubes. One is for nourishment and the other, which goes into your small intestine, is to return "stuff."

This morning we were told that you are now not so much in coma as you are deeply sedated. Where the dividing line is no one really knows. The hope is that very soon the methadone treatment will begin and you'll be awakened. Your lungs still are healing but, as we were told, you're getting better and better—the last two days really have amazed everyone.

I received an email this morning from a graduate student at Brigham Young asking if I would be teaching my course this term. I need to get back to Salt Lake. So many things have been let go. Yesterday, by the way, Aunt Tammy went to the house and found Bill Barnes cutting the lawn. Very kind. After speaking with the nurses this morning we were told that it probably would be all right for me to leave for a few days, that waking up takes quite a long time. My concern is that I want to be here when you awaken. Missing this moment would be like missing your birth.

> *Memory (age 18, May): "Last night Adam came home from bike riding with his friend James feeling pretty lousy. He'd taken a spill and landed hard with his chest on his handle bars. He felt badly enough that he couldn't lift his bike out of the van. He said he'd be all right [although] he was having difficulty breathing and really hurt. A few minutes before 8 p.m. we took him to the emergency room and tests began. He threw up a few times, which says something about how much he hurt. X-rays were taken which revealed that no bones were broken. A CAT-scan was done and something showed up on his liver, a 'gouge,' as one nurse put it. Fortunately, the sack around the liver hadn't broken (as of several minutes ago, hasn't), which means that blood isn't escaping into his body. The surgeon we met with last night said that just a few years ago the procedure was to immediately do surgery. Now, it is to wait and see what happens. Surgery, apparently, often does not go well. About 2 a.m. Adam was put into Intensive Care. Now, we wait."*

Becoming "Lighter"

September 5.

Dear Family and Friends,

It was a stable and quiet day for Adam. Some eye movement but mostly just the steady sound of machine-driven inhaling and exhaling. Adam is still critical, still unconscious, still breathing through a tube, but stable.

Today is the 24th day since your accident. It is 11:54 a.m. California time, September 5.

Dear Adam:

We understand that it is going to take several days for you to wake up. Before this happens you must be weaned from Morphine, the LICOX line in your head that measures brain oxygen has to be removed, and your oxygen levels (percentage of oxygen you are breathing) need to be near normal (28 percent. Right now you are at 60 percent—which is down from 70 yesterday). So, there is still a ways to go. Your mother and I both want to be present when you awaken. Missing this is unthinkable.

You look good, really good, and seeing your handsome face warms us. As we went into your room this morning we were told that there has been a discussion about what to do with your beard. Linda, the nurse you had yesterday, insisted that you not be clean shaven. Kirby and your mother agreed. Apparently there is a difference of opinion. That this would be an issue shows how far you have come.

4:15 p.m., California time, September 6.

Dear Adam:

Today you tried and tried to open your eyes with all sorts of encouragement from Rachel, your mother, and Kirby. Rachel actually recorded one of your efforts on her phone. Your mother cried. You blinked many times. Working very hard, afterwards you shivered. Then, you went deeper into unconsciousness. Apparently becoming "lighter" and then slipping deeper into unconsciousness, back and forth, is the typical pattern. Slowly the morphine dose is being cut in anticipation of beginning methadone treatment. We were told that Monday your head tubes will be removed.

As I write you are rather hot, hotter than a couple of hours ago. The CAT scan done this morning around 10:30 a.m. didn't show any infection in your torso, so that's very good. Your liver remains swollen but we were told the swelling is reducing. I should have mentioned yesterday that the blue plastic cooling devices that you have had on your torso and legs were removed. On Tuesdays and Saturdays your bandages are changed so today Rachel got to see (and photograph) your exposed head. I was in the room when the dressing on your stomach was changed. You are going to have a huge scar along with some "bullet" wounds. Maybe these body marks will satiate any desire you have had for a tattoo. I'd guess getting back your six pack is going to be very difficult. The sides of the wound, that I'd guess to be closer to nine than to eight inches long, are kept together by retractive sutures, long sutures that run through light brown plastic tubes that are knotted through a hole in the middle so the sides can be pulled in. The two tubes enter/exit your body near the incision a bit like a Cyborg from Star Trek.

Manny, age 30 or 31 and who has the "room" next to yours, has not had a good day. His family has been told that it is highly unlikely he will survive. He was badly beaten at a party. Hard to believe. A small artery in his neck has a leak that cannot be fixed. Even the attempt will likely produce a stroke that will kill him.

September 7.

Dear Family and Friends,

Mostly a quiet day. Why mostly? Unconsciousness is a matter of degrees and as Adam becomes "lighter" (more nearly conscious) he responds to various stimuli. Music is important, we've been told, and we sing to him and play recorded music, mostly his own. There are other forms of stimulation, one might think of them as irritants, to which he reacts: Rachel, Dawn Ann, Kirby and Michelle got very excited as Adam showed signs of responding to their loud pleas to move. "Adam," they commanded, "OPEN YOU EYES!" "Come on, Buddy, open your eyes"! Despite being deeply drugged and very tired he did, multiple times, do as commanded. Then, seeming exhausted, he would drift into deeper unconsciousness. Twice today, when Michelle pinched his chest, right then left side, he raised an arm in response. While his movement was lethargic it was also purposeful.

A Place of Sadness, a Place of Joy

September 7, 12:44 p.m. California time. Day 26.

Dear Adam:

Last night when we said "good night" (perhaps 8:20 p.m.) your numbers had dipped a bit, the fever was back, and your heart rate was up. Florence, the no nonsense nurse, said not to worry, urged us to let you rest, and, in effect, told us to go home. Before church at my urging your mother phoned to see how you were doing. Good news. Right now your numbers are 65 percent pure oxygen, which is up, your PEEP rate is 10, respiratory rate is 15 (this is why the oxygen level is up. Every number indicates a process that interacts with every other process—change one, change them all. Fifteen is the set rate. You've actually been as high as 24, I think. You are breathing quite often on your own, so your respiratory rate is actually higher than 15). Your Tidal Volume is 600 (the volume of air inspired or expired in a normal breath). This is somewhat low but allows you to breath more easily on your own. You are sweating and still hot to the touch. You've been given Tylenol and have ice packs made of surgical gloves in various places on your body. When I asked again about the fever I was told that it's common, that it takes the brain some time to reset body temperature. Also, being weaned from morphine may make you sweat. Yesterday the morphine setting was 4, today it is 3.5. Two is the magic number for starting methadone treatment. So, Adam, you are doing well for an addict!

Driving to the hospital is easier now than it has been although both Kirby and I get queasy feelings. She's also a worrier (and, your mother says, a "bolter"—she runs when you open your eyes). Waking up in the morning is also easier for me but remains a chore, even though I know where I am there is still just a hint of disbelief about what has happened. Then, too, waking up in someone else's home is a bit disorienting. Walking into the

SICU area I cannot wait to get into your room to see you and check the numbers. While I trust the nurses, seeing you and watching you breath is comforting.

When we walked into the waiting room today Manny's brother was sleeping on one of the chair beds as was Clio, a flamboyant woman and now friend whose husband, Elliot, is in SICU. Manny's family from New Mexico has gathered. While visiting you I looked at the numbers on the monitors in Manny's room; not good. If he survives I would guess he will be in a vegetative state. Karen, who has been here two weeks longer than you, said her first word two days ago: "okay." Susan, Karen's schoolteacher partner, was thrilled, and, beaming, spread the good news—It's good news for everyone. Elliot, now having had about a dozen surgeries bravely endures as does Tom. Richardo, a young Mexican, also had surgery. His mother greeted us as we walked into the SICU this morning. This is a place of such deep sadness and in this sadness people of radically different backgrounds and cultures bond, if but briefly. It is also a place of incredible joy.

9:55 a.m. California time, September 8.

Dear Adam:

You look great this morning although your head is in a crazy, awkward position. As weak as you are, I wonder if your head is going to fall off. You are not sweating like you were last night nor do you seem to have a fever—you were like a salt lick (Rachel kissed you and wiped her lips afterward, which I guess means she isn't bovine). We were told that the sweating continued throughout the night and that your heart rate was high as well, signs of morphine withdrawal. This, Heather, your young, tanned, California surfer nurse, said is called the "storm." At 6 a.m. this morning you were started on methadone, which settled you.

Sometime today the intracranial probe (LICOX) that measures brain oxygenation will be removed from your head. I had imagined something quite different from what it is—a small hole with a threaded connector screwed into the skull and thin wires. (We were just told that this will happen tomorrow, not today).

Last night your nurse, Florence, came into the waiting room about 7:30, much before the usual time visitors are allowed in to visit (7 to 8 p.m. is shift change). She said that we were welcome to come and visit you. She said she felt badly that last night she had been abrupt and had scurried us away. She said that she was concerned about your blood pressure and there was work she needed to do to get you where she wanted you. Then, she remarked, of all the patients she has had she feels most invested in and connected to you. She has been with you from the beginning and has come to love you and the family. She said that she "knew" from the beginning that you would be all right, but that you had given everyone a run for the money. You've worried her. (An aside: Dave's wife told me that every day after work he has come home and "talked about Adam". We got to meet her the other day, and she met you. Soon she and Dave will be parents for the first time).

Update: 12:30: We just met with Dr. Chang who removed several mucus plugs from your lungs. You are having some difficulty. There is concern about infection.

Dear Adam:

It is 4 a.m., Utah time, September 9. I haven't been able to sleep, but this isn't unusual.

I caught a 3:25 p.m. flight out of John Wayne Airport yesterday. Getting to the airport proved pretty stressful and not just because this was my first (our first) time away from you. We missed the 405 turn off and stayed on Interstate 5 until your mom realized we were heading in the wrong direction. I was getting pretty nervous which added to her and Rachel's stress. She took an exit and ran into an Albertson's, got directions, ran back, and off we went. From the terminal I phoned and spoke with Rachel who said "Mom had a meltdown." Being apart is very difficult. Although my sleeping has been fitful since we've been in California, having her nearby, hearing her breath, turn, go to the bathroom, is comforting.

Joshua and Vorn picked me up at the airport and we met Seth at Crown Burger to eat. On the way I told them that since I had written the update you had had a pretty difficult time, hitting what Dr. Chang called a "bump." Fever with indeterminate causes, complete with dripping sweat, difficulty processing oxygen (you were back on 100 percent oxygen) and higher PEEP numbers. Your incision was checked as were the tubes as possible sources of infection. Not there. Plans were made for a CAT scan of your head to see if you have sinusitis. This will presumably take place today. I didn't want to worry anyone, so I tried to not sound overly concerned.

I wasn't hungry but ate a hamburger.

Unplugged

Dear Adam:

Today is day 29. Your mother and I spoke earlier. The tubes have been removed from your head and you are wearing a meshed cap of some sort. She says you had a great night. The tubes were removed last night as Dr. Massoudi was called in because of Manny's worsening condition. Before he left, Shawn, your night nurse, urged him to remove the tubes, and he did. As I write, Manny apparently has been taken off life support. Your mother said that it can take up to 17 hours to die. So senseless. So sad. Thirty-one years old. I wonder who your next roommate will be. Several times I stood at the wall where your room and Manny's meet and watched him, thinking about the journey we have traveled.

You were shaved and now have a "soul patch" (a patch of hair beneath your lower lip). You probably won't like it. Also, you are passing gas—something you always liked doing when others were around (or so it seemed to me). As your mother and I spoke, I could hear Rachel's laughter in the background, which is a wonderful sound. I wonder what Rachel would think if she could see me—she'd probably scream. I had some pre-cancerous marks removed from my face yesterday morning, 22 of them, and it's not a pretty sight!

September 11—7th anniversary of the attack on the Pentagon and New York. Day 30.

It's 4:36 California time, Thursday.

Dear Adam:

I returned to California today from Salt Lake, arriving about noon at the John Wayne Airport.

Walking into your room was exciting. You are shaved, pale, the hair on your head is about one inch long—the scar on the right side of your head is impressive but when your hair grows out it won't be seen—and you are thin, really very thin, despite having a bloated torso. You are sweating great drops (part of being weaned from morphine). Yesterday you had gas—sufficient, I guess, to single-handedly increase America's energy reserves.

Seeing you this afternoon was wonderful. It's you, really you, just not the energetic you that I know. You opened your eyes and did your very best to keep them open as I talked to you. I don't know if you recognized my voice or not and I simply couldn't do what your mother urged me to do, talk "loud." Your eyes are expressionless and glazed, but clearly there is much going on inside your head despite still being drugged. You are getting closer to consciousness. Your mother and I wiped your face and head and then applied wet cloths to help cool you.

September 11.

Dear Family and Friends,

While sitting outside the SICU this afternoon, the seldom used fire-code escape door swung suddenly open and Michelle, Adam's nurse, appeared. Seeing us she called out, "Do you want to see inside Adam's lungs?" Both Dawn Ann and I were up in a flash, around the separating wall, and through the doorway. Dr. Chang was conducting a bronche to remove mucus plugs blocking the passage of air. Rachel had been taking a picture when Dr. Chang asked if she wanted to take a look through the scope. She did. Dave said, "Adam's Dad would love to see this." After we got to Adam's bedside, smiling, Dr. Chang held the scope for each of us to see—left lung, lower lobe—I looked, but given my infinite gradation glasses, I couldn't see anything. Still, I got to look.

It is 1:20 California time, Friday, September 12.

Dear Adam:

Last night, before we left, the A line was removed from your right arm and the staples were removed from the incision on your stomach. Michelle removed your staples with the able assistance of Kirby and Rachel, each of whom removed one. When they were all removed part of your incision, perhaps one inch long, opened, exposing just a bit of your innards. Michelle put out a call and one of the physicians came, cleaned the wound, and taped the two sides together. The rest of the wound was strengthened with surgical tape. Mom and I were told you had a blood clot and when the staples were removed the pressure of the clot opened the wound. Yesterday the sedative you were taking, Ativan, was stopped and sometime last night or this morning the morphine was also stopped. The methadone you are taking keeps you asleep, what seems to be a restful sleep although you continue to sweat mostly about your head. But, your temperature is normal.

You have two pressure ulcers, one on the top of your left foot (where a line had been) and another, found yesterday, on your throat beneath the right side of the trache. These were documented and photographed. Apparently this procedure is in effect because a rich kid and meth addict without insurance died in the unit. The family sued the hospital and won a large settlement because he had such a wound. Unbelievable. Taking a picture of the ulcer beneath the trache was quite a task, requiring two sets of hands— at one point including Kirby's. This was found, by the way, by Michelle as she was removing the stitches in your trache, put there as a preventative measure to make certain it stays in place. A white collar with Velcro ends now holds it firmly in place.

You received a new next door neighbor last night, your fifth, I think, a 97 year-old woman. She replaces Manny. Dave wondered why she was in the SICU since, as he said, there are so many bugs in the place that it's probably more dangerous for her to be in a hospital than anywhere else.

September 13.

Dear Family and Friends,

This morning Dr. Massoudi visited Adam and checked his eyes, reporting that his "pupils are briskly reactive...that's good." He went on to say that there are "signs" since Adam's last CAT scan of healing in the brain. Pausing, he then added, "If you open a neurosurgery text, Adam has had the full course. There is nothing, [no treatment, no medication], he hasn't had." Adam has never been one to do anything half way.

Shortly after Dr. Massoudi departed another physician stopped by and listened to Adam's lungs. Looking at all the pictures posted on the walls of Adam he remarked, "It looks like he's a real hell raiser. We've got to get him back so he can raise some more hell."

Memory (age 3, December): "A couple of weeks ago we received your preschool evaluation. You will be pleased to know that you were generally assessed to be 'very weak' by your teachers. The reason for the assessment is that you are something of a rebel and Montessori teachers don't like rebels at all, my dear, even three-year-old rebels. You have a fierce independence that gets in the way of you doing what you are told. Some examples: until recently you thought every school activity naturally, and normally, concluded with a visit to the 'time out' area—Adam, 'we pick up after ourselves, don't we?' 'Yes, and then we have time out.' Your mom told me you were spending lots of time in time out [recently] because you refused to put things away and lead a 'bat man' revolt. I asked what that was and she said you had some of the kids running around and jumping off of tables."

Memory (age 8, December): "'Adam, I'm going to school with you today to make certain you behave.' 'All day?' 'A chunk of it.' 'Gall, that's a long time...' 'Are you going to start doing your work?' 'I don't know. Sometimes it's hard to be good, you know.'"

September 13, 3:20 California time.

Dear Adam:

You are having mostly a very good day. You are off the morphine. You are still sweating some and your breathing is a bit labored but you are doing well. Until you were given methadone this morning, you kept your eyes open quite a lot—not quite responsive but not wholly elsewhere. Once the methadone begins to work you close your eyes and sleep. Kirby reported that while holding your hand she felt your fingers tighten (this was before receiving the methadone). We understand that it will take days for you to be fully weaned from morphine and then methadone, and it's not a pretty sight, I'm afraid. Again, your mother and I did our version of physical therapy with you, working your fingers, hands, arms, elbows and shoulders as well as your feet, ankles, knees and hips. Soon, I hope, we'll be formally taught just what to do and how to do it.

Another sign of your growing strength is that only one nurse has been assigned to you and your elderly neighbor.

Day 33. September 14, 3:22 p.m., California time.

Dear Adam:

When we arrived today after attending church we were greeted by a feverish son. Barry, your nurse, was preparing to remove your PICC line (peripherally inserted central catheter) and insert another line, hypothesizing the PICC was the source of a possible infection. You were given Tylenol, which dropped your temperature quickly. Later he turned a fan on to further cool you. Apparently last night you tried to pull off some of your lines and so your left arm is restrained but not the right. Don't ask me why the difference. You look good. You keep your eyes open quite a bit but you are still heavily drugged with Methadone, and very sleepy. Also you are rocking very slowly side to side which helps your lungs. We've been told it will take about two weeks—and this is a rough estimate—for weaning to be complete. Occasionally you frown, revealing a very sad face.

Last night you got another new neighbor—your sixth, I think. Some patients pass through very quickly. Bobby, 61 years-old, broke his neck surfing. His family has joined us in the waiting room. Lots of sadness. We haven't heard anything about Tom today although considerable effort went into getting Dee to leave for lunch. Not a good sign. Last night a decision was made that what happens is meant to be. Dee said, "I am at peace with the decision." I believe this means there will be no more extraordinary efforts to keep Tom alive.

There is now a regular hospital bed waiting next to the foot of your $35-40,000 rocking and rolling bed. Barry says that he'll move you into it sometime today and that is good news. You'll be much more comfortable in a regular bed. We don't know when you will be moved to another room, but we hope soon. When you are moved, therapy will begin, slowly at first.

September 15.

Dear Family and Friends,

For four hours this morning Adam has been breathing on his own. This is a huge positive step. In a few minutes he will be given a dose of Methadone and since he is already very tired from breathing unassisted a long and deep sleep should follow.

About 2:30 today Adam was holding Rachel and Dawn Ann's hands and staring at them. Steve, one of the nurses, asked Adam to nod his head if he knew they were there. In response, Adam nodded his head "yes," and raised his eyebrows. He was squeezing their hands, not wanting them to go. He also moved his toes and feet on command.

Adam's neighbor, Bobby, just passed away. A nurse mentioned that he was an organ donor, commenting on his and his family's generosity. Shortly after hearing this news, Brahm's Lullaby began playing over the hospital sound system, signaling a child has just been born.

September 16.

Dear Family and Friends,

Prepare yourself, dear reader, for another bit of good news. Adam is breathing on his own. The respirator has been removed. In the new room there is an oxygen hose that comes out of a connection in the wall. From this hose oxygen flows but unlike a respirator it does so without forcing a breath, breathing is the patient's responsibility. This is a big step forward.

Awakenings

Thursday, September 18, Day 37, 4 p.m., California time.

Dear Adam:

I returned to California this morning after spending a couple of days in Salt Lake. Being away was very difficult. Each time your mother phoned she had something delightful to report. I am amazed at what you have accomplished in the past three days. Today while I was sitting down at the computer to write the Caringbridge update your friend Laura came by, and, seeing me, smiled and hugged me. She had been to room 16 to see you and you weren't there. I told her where you are, that you'd been moved to room 14. Just a few minutes ago, while I was writing, Rachel came into the waiting room to tell me that she had asked Laura to speak in Spanish to you and that you understood her.

Originally four points on your brain were identified as seriously damaged, called "strokes," a fearsome word—you've now given signs that two of those areas, including comprehension, may not be as damaged as was feared. A miracle.

Right now you are very frustrated, and keep trying to pull out the oxygen tube, and we keep trying to get you to leave it alone. You just pooped and Heather and Michelle are cleaning you up. This must be so very difficult for you. It's hard to watch you suffer.

> *Memory (Age 22, Family Christmas Letter): Adam returned home in early November from his two-year church service in Southern California. He's now fluent in Spanish, and seems to think he's a Latin. Since returning home he's gotten registered for school and shows faint signs of starting to think about the future. He loved his*

service and made many wonderful friends. It's fun to once again have the house filled with Adam's music although sometimes a stomp or two [on the floor] is necessary to get him to turn down his amplifier downstairs.

Chin to Chest: Therapy Begins

September 18.

Dear Family and Friends,

Two physical therapy sessions today. The first involved moving Adam's hands and arms. While holding the therapist's hand he twisted his wrists and lifted his hands from the elbow. The therapist was pleased Adam could do 10 repetitions. Later, at noon, two physical therapists with the help of a nurse, disconnected Adam from most of the tubes and wires and helped him sit on the edge of the bed for 10 minutes, swaying, teetering. He sat, wearing his new, white, helmet, chin resting on his chest. Heads are heavy. He's incredibly weak, like a "baby" one therapist said.

Cognitive functions: We were told that he currently is at a level four: Level (1), no response; (2) generalized response; (3), localized response; (4), confused and agitated; (5) confused and inappropriate. Descriptors for level four include: being very confused and frightened, not understanding what he feels or what is happening around him, overreacting to what he sees, hears, or feels by hitting, screaming, using abusive language, or thrashing about, not paying attention or be able to concentrate for a few seconds. Based on what the first physical therapist told us this morning, it's likely he isn't at level four. (We don't know what to make of this scale which doesn't seem helpful at all)

> *Memory (age two, October): "You've now taken to a new way of life: You see yourself as a clown and engage in vigorous pretend acts of juggling—arms stiff and moving rapidly, eyes skyward, and mouth smiling... Last evening, as we prepared for bed, you threw a terrible fit when Joshua reached over and grabbed your arm while juggling. One of the pretend balls got away from you. You actually tried to juggle*

two Hot Wheels tires, but failed—probably the only thing athletically you cannot do. Between pretend games of baseball, running around the dinner table over and over again, juggling, and engaging in slow motion movements, you are a busy little fellow. As Aunt Tammy puts it, you are 'wild.'"

3:32 p.m., Friday, September 19, California time, Day 38.

Dear Adam:

I don't know why I hadn't thought about you needing to learn to speak again, but I didn't. The small muscles of the body take a hammering from five plus weeks of inactivity. Your therapist asked you to open your mouth a couple of times, which you did, barely. Slowly, ever so slowly, your mother and I are coming to appreciate the challenges that await us. It is difficult to imagine you actually eating and chewing something, which will be important to you gaining the energy you will need for physical therapy. We are hoping and praying that every ounce of your famed stubbornness will come into play, that you will take on the challenge of retraining your body with the same level of intensity you demonstrated when learning to play soccer or the guitar or to speak Spanish.

Rachel just came into the waiting room where I am writing this to tell me that you got angry because she wouldn't help you get up and out of bed, flipped her off, and tossed her from the room. (Level 4 behavior? Maybe there is something to these levels after all). "Oh, Adam, that's mean," she said, leaving (thinking it's funny). You are so frustrated, and we don't blame you. It's great you could flip her off!

Saturday, September 20. 4 p.m., California time.

Dear Family and Friends:

Today we were struggling to communicate with Adam, and Bob asked the nurses if we could try writing. Adam was moved toward a sitting position and Linda brought in a clipboard and some paper. Writing in a very wobbly and wandering script, we could make out two, and just maybe three, words: "I need...help." Yes he does. Adam also wrote "legs," which have been bothering him.

September 20.

Dear Adam:

Today Linda, your nurse, promised you that you would be home by Thanksgiving. She was trying to be encouraging but I fear if you thought about what she said, you are looking at another 9 weeks here. I hope she is wrong but suspect she is right. I'd like us to leave sooner. While you have made wonderful progress, it is clear that it is going to take a long time and a lot of work for your body to get to where it needs to be for you to be transferred home. Your left side is especially weak. Movement is difficult. Today on Caringbridge I wrote about you using your right hand to dip a swab and suck the water out. It is difficult for you to do this, find the cup to dip the swab to "drink" and then to find your mouth. This said, I'm thrilled you can do it at all. It's wonderful. I should probably mention that you place the swab in front of your teeth which must feel good to the gums.

Linda, by the way, is loud. Today she was chatting with your mother and the girls when you let her know—and them know—they were being too loud, this time signaling with your hand and arm to lower the volume. They got the message, and Linda left, her story unfinished.

September 21.

Dear Family and Friends,

Last night Adam was pretty funny, although he did not mean to be. He insisted that we put the shoes on his feet that his brother, Seth, designed and gave to him. We didn't have any socks for him to wear, so we used those thick, non-slip, blue-gray, hospital sock-shoes. It's not easy to get shoes over non-slip sock-soles. Once wearing the shoes he was very pleased, but thought this meant that he could leave the hospital, a first step toward running away. Not so. He wore the shoes for a couple of hours perhaps hoping we would turn our heads and he could dash. (Unfortunately, for Adam, dashing requires standing up and right now he can't long sit on his own without tipping over).

When we arrived at the hospital today a "Passy-Muir" valve had been placed on the trache which, according to a product advertisement, offers patients a "step toward independence and dignity through speech." For us, what this means is that we can hear Adam groaning, and he groans and groans—he did say "go" (meaning "leave") today.

Chewbacca Bellows

Sunday, September 21, 6:05, California time.

Dear Adam:

This evening our new Mission Hospital friend, Diana, Peter and Sue Mordin's daughter (Peter and Sue are from South Africa and are dear friends of Karen and Susan's), brought a white board and markers for you. This is a great improvement over using paper and pencil to communicate since the markers are easier to handle when writing. Your first words on the board were, referring to your nurse, "That guy doesn't help." Hmmm.

Dr. Chang dropped by about 5:50 this evening, saying you are doing great. The valve you have on the trache will enable you to speak, but thus far you really haven't chosen to do so. He said that it takes a little time. With the valve you groan, moan, in effect complain. All of this, mind you, is understandable. While I was rubbing your left leg a few minutes ago you let out a real strong complaint and a look of pain, indicating, I believe, a cramp.

Last night you were miserable, and it seemed as though you had gas. Tom, the nurse today, suggested you were plugged up. In any case, Linda ordered "the girls" out. You wanted me to stay and I did for quite some time, until a bit after seven p.m. I held your hand, sang to you, and you settled down and fell asleep.

Monday, September 22, noon, California time.

Dear Adam:

Earlier today you had three therapy sessions. While the speech therapist was working with you, she stopped and asked if you saw one or two of her. You indicated two. We are wondering if you are having double vision which would be yet another reason for keeping your eyes closed, not just being tired. The problem is your left eye.

Midnight tonight you get your last methadone dose. Hurray!

Your left side is really much weaker than your right but you actually urged the therapist to work the left side more. This is something that we talked about.

You are doing well but you cannot be moved to Acute Rehab, which involves three hours of therapy a day, until you are strong enough to benefit from the therapy. This means being able to sit up on your own. This said, each therapist today commented to us that you are making good progress. With the speech therapist you counted to five a couple of times and did some other positive things. We should have but neglected to mention to any of the therapists that you have written on a white board and that we are able to understand what you mean.

You now have a different trache, one that is smaller, and the valve has been removed. This trache facilitates speech and is an important step forward. I do not understand how all this works. I should mention that today you got so frustrated with my inability to understand you that you actually bellowed like Chewbacca, tilting your head back and letting out a wail. I felt badly, but we cannot let such feelings influence what we do for you or how we do them. We must be encouraging but also demanding.

A final word: you had me move the shoes Seth designed for Zuriick to your lap so you could look at and touch them. You are obviously very pleased to have them. Seth has asked if you'd also like a red pair. We asked, and you nodded that you did.

September 23. (Rachel writing)

Adam writing on the white board: "I need something to help me hold Rachel..." and that, "I need a blanket that will fit both of us."

I wrote him, "I love you." He wrote, "I love you too!" After writing this he took my hand in his and kissed it.

Several times he would ask, "Where is Mom?" "Where is Dad?" "Where is my family?"

I took a picture of Michelle and Adam together before moving out of room 14—the two of them smiled for the camera and afterwards embraced in a hug... Tenderly, Adam also pet Michelle's arm and flashed her the "I LOVE YOU" sign.

Before moving, Adam wrote to me, "I am nervous about my new room. You don't leave me." "I am a little scared."

Before leaving to gather our things for the 'sleepover' Adam wrote to Mom and me, "I am so thankful for you two." He was pleased when we told him that we were staying the night with him—he approved, flashing us the "thumbs up" sign.

While Kirby and I stood at his bedside Adam wrote, "Am I alive?" "Did they take my heart?" "They took Seth and my beating hearts out."

Upon our (Mom and my) return Adam wrote, "I missed you guys a lot. So don't leave again."

Adam has to wear a diaper for the night... He hates it. He wrote that it's, "Horrible." (Underlining that word).

Mom and I are going to spend the night tonight—we are in for a long night. But we are grateful that we can do this for Adam.

Rachel

Fears, Sleep Overs, Outings and Tests

September 24.

Dear Family and Friends,

Adam was very nervous about his new room and having a different medical team. Dawn Ann and Rachel decided to stay the night. Adam was very pleased with the idea of a sleep over, and gave a BIG thumbs up. He has his own room with an extra bed (no roommate). During the night Adam became very agitated and anxious, pulling at his IV line, trache, and bedding. He had to have a new IV line put in and the nurses restrained him which really upset him. Rachel and Dawn Ann spent the night trying to comfort Adam. At 12:30 a.m. the nurse gave him something to help him sleep...for three hours. Around 5:00 a.m. he desperately tried to get Dawn Ann to remove the restraints. She told him she couldn't, but that she loved him. He replied, speaking, "I love you, too." It was the first time Dawn Ann had heard Adam say those words since July.

September 25.

Dear Family and Friends,

This morning Adam went on a wheel chair journey, complete with a trailing oxygen tank (not quite a convoy but close). The entire journey took about an hour, start to finish. It's hard to believe how long it takes to get ready to travel: Being unplugged, dressed (including his new shoes with the purple soles and white crash helmet), then sitting on the edge of the bed, standing, ever so slowly, moving wobbly to a walker, shuffling a few steps and being positioned, then sitting down in the chair and reconnected to a portable oxygen tank. Makes me tired just to write the description. Our first stop was SICU, down a long hall and a left turn, where Adam was greeted, really lovingly swarmed, by many of the people who have cared for him. For Adam many of these were new faces, but they knew him—and parts of him in intimate ways. Daniel hugged us, and stooped down and gave Adam a bright smile and lots of encouragement. Having a bad taste in his mouth, Barry got Adam a "lemon swab" (Adam said it tasted like cotton). Looking ahead, Christine got him tooth paste and brushing sponges. Imagine how wonderful it is going to feel to have his teeth brushed. These are amazing and good people. From the SICU we traveled outside to the sitting area by the entryway where we have spent so many hours, waiting and waiting... and worrying.

While sitting at the computer to write this update, Kirby came into the room and urged me to come quickly, that Dr. Chang had arrived and was planning on removing the trache. We dashed to the room. Dr. Chang asked Adam if he wanted to remove the trache, and he did, perhaps thinking of all the miserable times he had been "bronched." Without hesitation, Adam pulled it out and handed it to Dr. Chang. Dawn Ann immediately asked if she could have it. "It's dirty," Dr. Chang said, but after hesitating gave it to her. She wants it to show her students. Never has a patient removed his own trache. Dawn Ann introduced Beverly, one of the nurses, to Adam, who has been with him from the beginning of his hospital stay. The first words he spoke since having the trache removed were, "Hi, Beverly." She was thrilled.

Memory (Age 5, February): "Today I walked into the kitchen and found you in a rocker with the kitchen stool upside down and in front of you. Your hands were on the rocker's arms. 'I'm handicapped,' you said. 'You are? Are you in a wheelchair?' 'Yes, it's remote control'."

10:32 a.m., California time, Day 45, September 26.

Dear Adam:

I returned to California yesterday morning after a pretty intense few days in Salt Lake. Finding black mold in the basement bathroom, Tuesday morning

I discovered the water heater had been leaking. I spent the day running around like mad (5 or 6 trips to the hardware store after a trip to Lowes and Home Depot to purchase a water heater), spending a small fortune, but by about 5:30 I had finished installing a new water heater and cold water filter except for a few little things that I finished up late Wednesday night. I didn't sleep much.

Wednesday was busy at work. After class I chatted with Josh who said that he had something that he wanted me to take to you and said that I should drop by the house and get it and have some lasagne with him and Vorn. When I arrived, sometime after 8:00, Josh and Vorn had a wonderful dinner ready and Josh gave me a Led Zepplin buckle to give to you, a 1976 original, that he purchased. I gave it to you yesterday, and you were delighted.

When I arrived in California you were pleased to see me and I you. Your mother and Rachel had spent the night with you in the hospital and both were very tired. I spent last night so they got some sleep. Kirby came by after her class last night, sometime around 10:30 and stayed as you slept until I encouraged her to go home. She's a good person.

Everyone here is very optimistic that you are going to get back your physical abilities. Talking about this with you this morning was comforting. In fact, while you often tell people you don't want to talk any more, this time you wanted me to say more and more about how the brain works and how systems re-route themselves. I worked your legs and hands. The needle in your left arm makes exercising a little difficult. You also did some exercises on your own, which is very positive.

One of the trauma physicians came by this morning to check on you. As we talked, he laughingly said that "all of you here (referring to your mother, Rachel, and me) know more about [his] case than [I do]." He reviewed the "paperwork" on you, said everything looks great. He noted that your left is weaker than your right side and asked if you could move your extremities on your left side. You did. Watching you, he said you're going to get all of your strength back. Your mother just came by to tell me that the physical therapist is in your room and they have you up and walking, such as it is... seven steps.

Memory (age 13, February): "*Adam and I played a little one-on-one basketball at the [neighbor's house]. Our [little] court had snow on it. He made some incredible shots, including the game winner which was unbelievable, one of those only Michael Jordan makes coming in on the right side and spinning—but this time it was a short, little, white kid who put it down! He was so fun to watch. He was amazing, hitting shots from probably 25 feet out.*"

Memory (age 7, February): "*During our family activity we played Darth Daddy—yes, Darth Daddy has returned. (Kids wrestling with their dad) You and Rachel were hilarious. Both of you stripped to your underwear, yelled and growled and flexed your little sinewy muscles before attacking me. It was great fun although Rachel is a fragile warrior—and you just won't stop, wildman! Before leaving for school the next day you said, 'Daddy, did you like playing Darth Daddy last night?' 'Yes,' I said. 'I'm going to have Darth Daddy as my activity [next week].'*"

September 27, 5:57 p.m., California time.

Dear Adam:

We spent much of today waiting for an evaluation of your swallowing ability. Apparently Amanda, your speech therapist, left a message requesting a physician order the test but no test was ordered. So, tomorrow the test will be done. We're disappointed because once you pass this test you will be able to begin eating, actually eating, real food and get closer to having the feeding tube removed. You might have complained, but you did not. You remain remarkably appreciative, expressing thanks to everyone in a surreal, almost child-like way. It takes a lot of energy to speak, so you tend to avoid speaking except when a "thank you" is called for. We, on the other hand, do our best to get you to talk. As I mentioned yesterday, coordinating breathing, vocal chord and lip action, is very complicated and tiring. Today the gauze was removed that covered the place—I almost said "hole", but it isn't a hole anymore—where your trache was. This is referred to as a sort of badge of honor. You'll have a small scar.

About 15 minutes ago we returned from one of our hospital outings, this one down and around the hallways, and then outside where what had been a very hot day was cooled by a sweet breeze. You enjoyed yourself. Barbara, the rehab person, showed Mom and me how to recline the wheel chair, which made sitting more comfortable for you. Getting ready for this trip involved you walking across your room in the walker and to the wheel chair—taking several labored steps. You obviously had to think carefully about walking, especially getting your left leg to move in front of your right. Returning to your bed after the journey, the nurse, Richard, had you do more walking, this time moving your feet while sitting in the wheel chair to position the chair in just the right place so you could be shifted into bed with relative ease. Richard did a very nice job. On your part, you worked hard to hold your head up and to help get ready for the trip and your return, including putting your hands on Richard's shoulders and helping him lift you out of the wheel chair.

Earlier in the day a bully nurse's aide worked with you, basically pushing you around, insisting you shouldn't wear pants (too inconvenient for him, I'd guess) and giving your mother grief when she told him that today was the first day you hadn't been wearing pants, that you liked to wear them. What precipitated the confrontation is that while trying to pee you spilled. He was quite irritated. I do not think he had any idea who he was dealing with. Your mother told Richard, who likely is responsible for supervising him, that she didn't want him in your room again. And he wasn't. You've not said an unkind thing about anyone since we have been here, but you said of this fellow, "He's a jerk." Yup.

Sometime this afternoon a little confrontation took place. Using the walker, which is on wheels, Kirby hoisted herself up by her elbows while Rachel pushed her around for a ride. They then switched positions. Seeing this activity you angrily flipped them off, saying, "That's hard for me!" You were upset. Rachel and Kirby were both upset as well about hurting your feelings. Your mother said that you really felt badly afterwards about what you had done.

Day 47. September 28, 7:50 a.m. California time.

Dear Adam:

I explained to you that I needed to go to the waiting room for a moment. You looked at me and said, "hurry." I will. Quite the night, Adam. I'll describe for me the busiest sequence, running from about 3:45 a.m. to 4:20. You called to me. "I have to pee." I went to your bedside and you had your pants down and the pee-bottle positioned. (I had placed one bottle on each side of the bed on the rails) While waiting the nurse's aide came by to do the 4 a.m. check. I waited until you were finished urinating, got you a paper towel to do a little clean-up, and took the bottle and set it by the sink, making a point of telling the aide, who was then doing whatever he needed to do for you, where the bottle was. After picking up the paper towel and tossing it away, I went back to bed. A few minutes later you called, this time by a kind of groaning sigh, a signal. I know you want me when the signals get a bit louder and more frequent. I got to your bedside and you wanted to be moved up in the bed. Already you had lowered the bed and flattened it. Using your right arm, you grabbed hold of the headboard and together we moved you. I did some rearranging, as directed, and went back to bed. You began making your summoning noise again. So, I got up and asked if you were all right. You asked, "How much did I pee?" I showed you. "Did you tell the nurse?" (A report is to be made of when you pee and how much). I explained that I put the pee-bottle by the sink and told the aide. Another summons. You were hot and wanted the fan moved. I moved it, rearranged the sheet that had been covering you, and asked if you wanted a cool wash cloth. You did, so I got one which you took and did a bit of wiping of your face and chest. I went back to bed. Then, you were thirsty. I went down the hallway and got some ice and put some water in a cup. Not wanting to turn on a light, I couldn't find one of the pink sponges so we used one of the tooth brushing sponges for dipping. "I am really thirsty," you said. And you were. I held the cup as you swished the sponge about with your right hand and sucked the water out. A bit more rearranging. Back to bed. More noises. I checked on you. You wanted to be turned. It took me a while to understand what you wanted. You wanted to be more on your side. So, I helped you get rearranged. Back to bed. You quieted and I walked to the SICU waiting room thinking I'd type this up. The room was dark and three of Mr. Han's family members were sleeping. I went back to bed. Now, as I said, this was my most busy period with you. All along the way you made a point of saying "thank you." I was glad to help.

September 28.

Dear Family and Friends,

Although quite nervous, this afternoon Adam "passed" the swallowing evaluation. He was fed barium-laced stuff of different consistencies while being x-rayed. After the test Adam asked if he could have a root beer. Sadly, right now the liquids he's allowed to drink must be thick or thickened (a process that involves mixing a chemical of some kind into the liquid). Adam does not like the result so he's still sucking a pink sponge stick when he wants a cold drink of water.

As I write, Adam is eating his first "normal meal" since August 12th. It's not entirely certain just what he is eating. We know that the steak-like thing is made of pureed pork, there is something green that might be made of green beans, and something else of indeterminate origin, something sort of yellow. There is also thickened milk and a thick fruit drink of some kind. Behind Adam, posted on the wall, is a yellow sheet of paper stating the "Swallow Guidelines:" "Nectar thick," "no thin liquids or ice," "no straws," "upright position," "90 degrees in chair or bed," "wait for swallow before next bite," "alternate foods with liquids," and "feed only when awake/alert." Personally, I like the last one since I very much enjoy eating while asleep. Adam's nurse stressed the guidelines, adding, "one bite at a time." And, we were told, "No questions while Adam eats" (an unwritten rule).

I've never thought of eating as particularly tiring, but Adam found it necessary to take a break and recline (remember the rule: "90 degrees in chair or bed") and rest. He's getting stronger.

Tomorrow will be a big day. Adam will be moved into Acute Rehab to begin an intensive program of therapy. We still have no sense of a time line but, as our friend Peter Mordin said today, unlike the first two stops this one has an "end point"—going home.

September 29. (Dawn Ann writing, a Caringbridge update)

Dear Family and Friends,

Today the speech therapist did an assessment and asked Adam to reply to questions with first thoughts. Question: "What is slippery when wet?" Answers: "A bike chain when its wet, ... The floor... Question: What can you eat that is frozen?" Answers: "Frozen yogurt, ice cream and those things, they are rectangular, brown, TOASTER STRUDELS!" My favorite was: Question: "What tastes better the next day?" Adam looked puzzled. He thought and thought. A hint: "Can you think of an Italian food?" "Pasta?" Then we laughed and Adam explained that he doesn't eat left overs. As his mother, I can attest to this fact.

Today Adam was moved to Acute Rehab.

Therapy, Therapists, and Wearing Down

Dear Adam:

Yesterday you moved to Acute Rehab.

Your affect has really been rather flat. To get a smile we've had to ask you for one and only recently has your smile looked like a real smile rather than a stiff, painful and toothy grimace. On Sunday, while listening to Blind Faith, which you think is the best band ever, you cracked a smile as you tapped your right hand on your thy and bounced your right foot in rhythm with the music. Also on Sunday, while someone was visiting, I commented on your eye-patch, which helps with the double vision. Without hesitation, you gave a pirate growl, "RRRRR." Good signs. Now, having pointed to these incidents, I should also mention that you have said a lot of very funny things but you are unaware they are funny. For example, the first words out of your mouth to Dr. Chang were, "I farted." There is an innocence in what you say, a matter-of-factness, of the sort slightly diminished people have who are unaware of social context and say just what comes to mind.

Last night Rachel stayed with you. I hope the night went well. Being in your new room, Room 102, probably was a bit disorienting. Today the hard work of rehab begins.

I saw Dr. Massoudi yesterday. Your mother refers to this meeting in the Caringbridge entry, when he said that you are the "miracle patient of the year," like an award winner. What she didn't say is that while we were talking she came up and mentioned your interest in his Ferarri—he said that he's looking forward to showing it to you.

During Dr. Chang's visit yesterday your mom gave him a dozen Paradise Bakery cookies, which he loves. He's been very kind and we trust him, completely. I was on a plane, so I missed this interaction. I guess the two of you had quite a chat about music, which included discussion of how guitars work, you noting that electric guitars are too sensitive for you to play right now given the difficulty of controlling your left hand. I got the impression that he was encouraging you to work at playing, even if your hand didn't yet cooperate.

> *Memory (age 19, June): "Your determination to learn to play the guitar is amazing. It's only been a year since you hurt [your liver] and in that year you have become a guitarist... Your mother goes nuts listening to you practice... Too bad Rachel and your mom have to sleep, else you'd probably get to do what you want, play all night."*

October 3, 4:37 pm, California time.

Dear Adam:

The meeting this morning with the various therapists, the social worker, neuropsychologist and an insurance person, was really rather depressing. Once out of the hospital our insurance will pay for a total of 25 occupational therapy sessions, no more. You are now getting about 6 sessions per day, which puts the insurance benefit into perspective. This makes no sense.

The neuropsychologist was rather smug and very irritating. She had a few notes in front of her as she spoke, undoubtedly made by others since she has never met you (although she dropped by for a visit today and stayed long enough to borrow a book and ask you a few questions). The one helpful point she made was that you need to recover yourself, a very difficult challenge. From my perspective, this is in part a narrative problem, of needing to recapture stories of self. She also made a big point of saying that you are not "retarded" but that developmentally you are like a "smart ten-year-old." You need, she said, to go through the same sort of stages you went through growing up, moving from childhood to adulthood—which includes slowly gaining in the ability to concentrate.

Here I should mention that your sense of humor shows occasional signs of returning even as you are battling depression. I so wish folks would stop asking you how you are and rather concentrate on what you can do now that you couldn't do even a few days ago—sit up without falling over; pushing with your legs as we slide you up in bed; and talking pretty clearly (although with a Forrest Gump quality).

Last night, by the way, eye patch in place, you watched part of the Vice Presidential debate, and enjoyed it immensely (you are an Obama fan). The part of your brain that was initially hammered includes the cerebellum, which accounts for your struggle with coordination (this is the ataxia problem you are facing, where your left hand and leg—and to a much smaller degree your right hand and leg—don't quite do what you want then you "overshoot" and "undershoot" as Kelly, your physical therapist said).

You picked up your guitar for a moment. We have been told that this isn't wise, that it's likely to increase your frustration. You do have some specific finger exercises, however. Balance and core body strength, we've been told, are foundational to all other physical activity, so that's the focus of most of your therapy right now.

You are able to help get yourself into and out of the wheel chair, which is significant progress, and you are taking a few more steps. The neuropsychologist said that a lot of our orientation to space comes through the joints, and this is also an important area of focus. She said, "with brain injuries [we go] from the bottom to the top."

I should also mention that you are eating real—grated but not pureed—food. Sadly, nothing tastes as it should.

We are concerned about the insurance issue, although I can't complain since we've been wonderfully blessed to have had you on our account at all.

Today has been a very difficult day for your mom. She has been in tears about Mr. Han, who is still alive but awaiting having his organs harvested. His is a wonderful family. As I write, Mrs. Han and her two daughters are sitting behind me. He was a painter and fell off a roof working. Also, you have been really down. Not only do you fixate on Eric Clapton, you talk frequently about getting out of this place and back home. We are concerned about the road ahead and what will be required of us...and of you. Mom commented to me that "at least" I get to go home and get away from here while she's trapped in the hospital. And she's tired.

Rachel is also very tired. Tomorrow she has a date with Matt, which is great. She perks up when speaking of him. Happily, some days ago my dean dropped by to tell me that he would support me in any way I need to enable us to help you recover. Your mother needs to get to Wasatch Elementary School and to work (the other day the teachers cleaned out her room so another teacher could move in) and she needs to begin taking endorsement classes for her new job as school librarian. Lots to do. Tomorrow is Tom's memorial service. This also weighs heavily. Lots of sadness right now.

> Medical memo: "The cerebellum (Latin for little brain) is a region of the brain that plays an important role in the integration of sensory perception, coordination and motor control. In order to coordinate motor control, there are many neural pathways linking the cerebellum with the cerebral motor cortex (which sends information to the muscles causing them to move) and the spinocerebellar tract (which provides proprioceptive feedback on the position of the body in space). The cerebellum integrates these pathways, like a train conductor, using the constant feedback on body position to fine-tune motor movements." [10]

Discouragement

October 5.

Dear Family and Friends,

Today we got Adam dressed, put him in his wheel chair, and went and visited his beloved car, a 2001 Escort, Desmond. Looking Desmond over Adam noticed someone had hit him. Given all the fancy cars in the parking lot Dawn Ann's response was, "I hope whoever hit the car and left did more damage to their car than to Adam's." We then visited the SICU and the nurses there. It's impossible to adequately say how wonderful these people are and how kind and good they have been to Adam and to us. Erik talked "Clapton" and guitar with Adam (when Adam was in coma Erik worked Adam's fingers in various chord patterns). Gil gave Adam encouraging words as did Alisha and Christine, among others.

Day 55, October 6, 10:10 a.m. California time.

Dear Adam:

This morning as we walked into the hospital we ran into Felipe, who had just visited you. He had a big smile on his face as he greeted us. As we chatted he said that you are the "sickest patient" he has ever cared for. By the way, he was one of the respiratory therapists who worked, and worked, on you during the most difficult of times for you and for us. He said that seeing you makes everything worthwhile, that you are "really amazing." I complimented him on his skill and hard work to which he said, it wasn't us, it was, and then he pointed upward, "Him." So many of the people in the SICU are people of faith, and for Felipe and others you have helped strengthen their faith and commitment to their work. On my part, I do not know how they do what they do. Rebecca, by the way, another of the respiratory therapists, visited you yesterday. So did Dr. Chang, who said that you are no longer his patient, that his was a social visit. It's amazing how my perception of him has changed. How hard it must be for physicians and nurses to have to give bad news to family members of critically ill patients. How in the world do they know what to say? Each of these people seems to gather energy from you and from your progress and in turn you gain strength.

Still, you are battling discouragement, although I should also note that you really came alive during our visit to SICU yesterday. Discouragement, as you remarked yesterday, certainly is "normal," but it will also destroy you. On your part, being fixated on getting home you are doing everything you are told to do—"whatever" is a word that you often use, a statement of being resigned, but not quite, to your state, of being totally in others' control and lacking agency. You try and try to defer decisions to others saying, "whatever you want" or "it doesn't matter", which is a bit worrisome. Your strong will asserted itself in your earlier battle for life, and now that will is needed perhaps more than ever.

When going home last night Kirby and I spoke. She wonders who you will be when you are back—so do we all.

There was a lot of tension between you and your mom yesterday. At one point she told you in no uncertain terms, and standing at the foot of your bed in her teacherly way, that your progress is in your hands, and that she, for one, isn't going to sit by and allow you to stay in bed and deteriorate further (noting that in your mind, yesterday, Sunday, was a day of rest). She mentioned the figure we've often heard, that for every day in bed it takes four to recover—you said she made that up. By happenstance, Chuck, the respiratory therapist from yesterday mentioned the same thing, but used the figure one to seven. This got your attention, which irritated your mother even further since apparently you were willing to believe Chuck but not her. We got you to eat pretty well, achieving the 75 percent needed to move toward getting the feeding tubes removed, and this required some pushing. Additionally, last night, when you said that you had to "pee," I responded by telling you that this meant we needed to walk to the bathroom, that you shouldn't use what you call your "pee cup." So, I got you sitting up, and began to get the wide cloth gait belt around your chest to help lift you (which worries you—if it slips it touches the tubes in your stomach, which must hurt) and then I remembered the feeding tube, which needed to be disconnected first. So, down you went and we called the nurse. Tube disconnected and flushed, up again, helmet and strap on, you and I edged our way to the bathroom with the nurse moving along slowly and attentively behind. With some help you did your business, cleaned up, and we again worked our way, misbehaving legs and all, back to the bed where you collapsed, exhausted. I was thrilled and got the tape measure that your friend Mark from the Children's Museum brought by and measured the distance—24 feet one way!

Tubes and Talking

October 6.

Dear Family and Friends,

Dawn Ann stayed with Adam last night. They had a good night, although he's becoming rather talkative (mostly about not very interesting things, like having his new $200 jeans cut off by the paramedics when he first fell and Clapton and more Clapton).

The tube issue came to a head today. Not knowing the rules, when Adam said he had to pee this morning, having done two therapy sessions, Bob said, "Let's walk to the bathroom," which they did last night. Helmet and gait belt in place, Bob in front, Rachel in back (Dawn Ann at Costco) we made our way to the bathroom, slowly, deliberately, awkwardly. While Adam did his business, Bob waited attentively, eyes averted, at the door. "I'm finished." Bob turned, gave Adam some wash cloths and wipes, and prepared to lift him on a three count. "I need the wheel chair," Adam said. Rachel brought it over and positioned it by the door. Now, we do not know what happened but Adam and Bob deny any culpability and neither one blames the other. "One, two, three..." Oops. Out popped the "G" (gastrointestinal) tube. The end of the G tube, the part inserted into Adam's body looks a bit like one of those plaster board metal fasteners that bends inward and expands as a screw is turned. Adam was stunned. Shocked. Bob was stupefied, then concerned. (When Dawn Ann returned she helpfully commented that she had been told that Adam should not be walking yet. No one told Bob nor Adam this. Probably a liability issue.) Double oops. With the tube out food leaked through the hole on Adam's lower stomach, about 3/8 inch in diameter, and ran downward onto his pants. Not good. "Rachel, call the nurse!" Breaking rules is one thing, getting caught is another. So, Bob covered up Adam and the two of them, shamefaced, waited.... Adam worrying. Bob doing some quick cleaning, the tube draped limply over the toilet paper dispenser. The nurse arrived, a fresh and thin tube was inserted and pushed deeper into the hole (it didn't exit, at least not to our knowledge, which was a relief), and we got Adam back to bed where some serious fretting began. Adam did NOT want the tube replaced. He reminded all who would listen that he had been eating 75 percent of the food at each of his meals for "days," the standard for being allowed to eat real food, not pureed, not grated. A bit of an exaggeration. Word was sent to get a trauma nurse to come and determine whether or not an attempt should be made at replacement; Adam's nurses were not allowed to make such important decisions. While nervously waiting, a therapist came by and did some work with Adam... And Adam worried and waited. Seeing Daniel from SICU walk through the door was a relief. Smiling as only Daniel can, he asked how Adam was doing, about how he was eating—three good days—told him he needs to keep "eating well," and covered the hole with gauze and tape saying it will close up on its own. Hugs followed. So, one tube left and Adam will be untethered, less Cyborg-like.

October 10, 12:10 p.m., Salt Lake time.

Dear Adam:

I'm writing now because you phoned this morning, which really amazed me. At first I didn't recognize your voice, and then I felt the joy of hearing you speak. You told me that your last tube had been removed about twenty minutes earlier and that all of the stuff on your stomach has been removed. I was thrilled. You said that you'd been told to be careful, at least for a day. You complained about being told that you needed to drink Ensure, saying that you worried it would leak out the hole in your stomach. Also, you mentioned that the hole from your "G" tube had already closed. Amazing. Such great news. We only spoke briefly because you had to leave for therapy.

Speaking of therapy: We have made arrangements for you to stay another week in the hospital. Your mother and I have been debating how to tell you, but we both think this is important for your recovery. Unfortunately, on the way home from the airport on Wednesday I mentioned to Seth that we were thinking about doing this and he, of course, told you. My fault. He said he thought he'd recovered when you acted surprised and disappointed by the news, Seth saying that he probably got the date wrong. Oh, well. So, we're now looking at October 28th rather than the 22nd to leave. This may not seem like a big deal, but you get six therapy sessions in the hospital each day. Originally, the idea of an extension was placed in my head by Perry, one of the therapists. Our action was based on the belief that once home you would only be covered for a total of 25 sessions. I found out, however, that our insurance will pay for the cost of Rehab Without Walls as long as you show signs of improvement, which is wonderful news. We understand that this program will provide about three hours of rehab six days a week at our house.

Oh, I should mention that last night Diann Weixler walked Layla. I bumped into her as I was leaving the house to get a longer gas line for the water heater, so we chatted. She said that your injury has really brought the entire neighborhood closer together, that everyone talks about you.

Tonight, Rachel and Kirby will be in charge. Be kind to them.

> *Medical memo: "Despite all the work and thinking done thus far, we still do not have a 'magic bullet' treatment that will cure any of the degenerative diseases, nor do we have an effective, universally accept clinical treatment for brain and spinal cord trauma (indeed, it is interesting to note that research on behavioral and functional recovery from brain damage is one of the least-funded areas of research sponsored by the National Institutes of Health and no funding in this area is provided by the National Science Foundation)."* [11]

Looking Ahead, Thinking of Home

Tuesday, October 14, and I'm still in Salt Lake.

Dear Adam:

Mom flew back to California yesterday morning, early, following her only visit to Utah. She was anxious to get back and to see you. While we were away, Saturday night Rachel wrote the Caringbridge entry, which was fabulous.

While here in Salt Lake your mother and her sisters worked their hearts out cleaning, getting the house ready in anticipation of your return—nothing inside really has been done in two months. Joshua and Vorn have taken care of the yard and animals.

Sunday your mother and I spoke in church. When I mentioned this to you, you were surprised to hear that you were the topic. It was exactly two months to the day of your accident when we spoke. Your mother had an outline and skillfully and with humor told stories. She did a great job. I read very brief excerpts from this journal and made a couple of points, that prayers are heard and miracles happen.

Lest I forget, here is a "thank you" note you wrote to be mailed to Mark and your friends at the Children's Museum. I just happened to notice it last night on the dresser. It is written in a very shaky hand, but it says a lot about where you are in your recovery. It reads:

"Dear Mark and museum people. Thank you so much for your support. I remember when you came by Mark. Sorry I was messed up & in SICU so I couldn't really talk or anything. Things have gotten a little better. I can talk now. In the therapy files they have written that I'm a smart-ass. I'll see you soon. Adam."

I love you, Adam. Dad

October 16.

Dear Family and Friends,

Beckie and Tammy (Dawn Ann's sisters) and Tammy's family, Dan and the kids, arrived from Utah today. It was a happy reunion that really perked up Adam.

October 18. Saturday.

Dear Family and Friends,

Another day of intensive therapy. When we arrived at the hospital this morning, after parking, we noticed a figure moving outside. It was Adam, in his walker. With help he worked his way up the wheel chair ramp toward the steps where we spent so many hours sitting, talking on the phone, and worrying during August, and then back down again toward the SICU entryway. Quite a sight to behold. "Keep your head up, Adam." [During therapy] and standing between parallel bars Adam and Bob kicked a soccer ball back and forth and Adam and Dawn Ann played catch, more or less. Activities like these sometimes frustrate Adam, but he complies knowing that the harder he works now the better he will be when at home. Near the parallel bars is an exit. Yesterday, while waiting to raise himself to the bars to practice walking, Adam looked at the door and said, "Don't put me by an exit, I might try to escape." We think he was joking.

October 19. It's 7:11 p.m. California time.

Dear Adam:

You are still slowly working on eating your salad that Heidi made—and you are being nice to Matt. While I was writing on Caringbridge your mother came into the waiting room to report that I have missed you performing the seizure that you have decided to have if Eric Clapton visits you (I wish Rachel never mentioned the letters I wrote to him about you asking for a note of encouragement—four of them. One already sent back as undeliverable. You say he lives in Ohio, so maybe I should have written a different sort of letter, something about the Buckeyes.) I'll have to finish this letter tomorrow in Salt Lake.

Today, the 20th, is John Dewey's 149th birthday. Your mother phoned me before I boarded my plane to say that you took a bath! Yes, yes!! This morning, before leaving, I watched as you did two of your therapy sessions. One involved taking a ball that weighed about 5 pounds and moving it about in different ways, lifting it over your head ten times, to the left and to the right ten times, and so on. You got beads of sweat on your nose, which says something about how exhausting the workout was. Holding the ball in both hands helps your balance and helps strengthen your left side; you favored the right on several of the exercises. In the earlier session you had to stand alone and take steps forward and backward and then side to side, alternating. You did very well. It was fun to watch. You know just about everyone's names and greet everyone. They, in turn, talk with you, ask how you are doing, and try and be encouraging.

Dr. Massoudi still has not visited, but word was sent that they'll do the bone flap replacement—a cranioplasty—surgery sometime early in November or December. This doesn't help us. We have no way of planning and if we are to bring you home and then return for the surgery we're looking at a lot of money to fly. Pretty discouraging.

Dear Family and Friends,

Tina, a therapist, taught Rachel and Dawn Ann how to walk with Adam, holding his gait belt, hand upward. She taught Adam and Rachel how to help Adam if he falls, he even did a fake fall, and then how to help him up. Just in case. No real falls yet.

Wednesday, October 22, day 71.

Dear Adam:

I'm in Salt Lake. Bone flap surgery has been scheduled for next Monday, the 27th, at 4 p.m. You'll spend a day in SICU and we're hoping you'll be discharged on the 29th or 30th. Lots to do.

I spent yesterday running around and trying to get things arranged for your return. Early in the morning I scheduled flights for Heidi, Kirby and Emmely to come to Salt Lake for Thanksgiving. I began checking on absentee voting and downloaded the forms needed. But, now that you'll be in Salt Lake on election day this isn't an issue. Next came setting up Rehab Without Walls. These folks were great and even called back later in the day to let me know that tomorrow, Thursday, someone will come to the hospital to assess your needs so that plans can be made for your care. We have a rehab physician, Dr. Ryser, who you will meet on December 11th but you'll start rehab well before then. Monday evening Vorn downloaded Social Security forms for me, so I need to check these out. I was told that hospitals have Medicaid help centers, so I went to LDS hospital only to be told that everything has been moved to another hospital. I then went to the old Holy Cross Hospital, where you were born, and there was told to go to the business office and ask for Nichol. Nichol gave me a form but didn't know anything about filling it out or what to do. So, I asked if there was a Medicaid center nearby. She didn't know and couldn't find an answer on the web, so she made a call. With address in hand—720 South,

2nd East—I continued my journey undaunted but slightly irritated.

I walked into the Workforce Services Building which was full of folks, people from all over the world. I walked up to one of the clerks and told her what I was doing and why and asked what I should do. She gave me the same form Nichol earlier had given me and, pointing to the south, said, "Fill this out" and mentioned it could also be filled out online. A young man came up to me while I was working on-line—I'd found the form—and asked what I was doing. I gave a quick description and, trying to be helpful, he messed with the computer and took me right back to where I started. I asked if there was any advantage to filling the form out online. He said it was a good idea because, pointing, I wouldn't have to stand in that line. I looked to my right, got his point, and went to work. Perhaps 20 minutes into things, a large woman came up to me and again I was asked what I was doing. Briefly I told her, my third report, but before finishing a women in a brightly colored dress sitting nearby interrupted. I waited and waited for her to finish talking. The large women really didn't want to listen to her or to me. She was in a hurry. Who knows why, but she did say when she walked away that she needed to get "back to work." I said that you were hurt in California...and I was then told, even before finishing the thought, well, that's California's responsibility. The large woman said, "I wouldn't even fill out the forms until you are in Utah" and then, she added, all that will happen is that any payment will be delayed. Moving away, she volunteered, "with all the recent cuts, you won't be getting any help anyway." I tried to hold her attention for a brief moment more to tell her that in California we were told that no help would be forthcoming because you weren't a resident. Catch-22. She left. I left. I now understand why lawyers get involved in such matters.

A Grim Facticity

Dear Adam:

A few minutes ago, after playing with your food, you got into your wheel chair and made a trip down the hallway. Your mom and I only knew you left when we heard the door close. We went to the door and saw you off down the hallway looking at the pictures of the various people who work in the Acute Rehab Unit. Your mother laughed. She knew what you were doing, or thought she knew. You didn't want to use a walker, so you thought a preemptive strike was in order and you went to rehab rather than having rehab come to you. She said that you were unhappy that in your last session you were made to walk the long way around, which tired you out.

I should mention that after rehab this morning, which involved tossing a ball against a thing like a small trampoline so that the ball bounces back for catching, you walked back to your room. On the way you needed to pause, and sometimes your left leg shook with fatigue. It is hard work. I should also mention that we've learned to let you do everything you can on your own. You are generally pretty insistent about doing so, which is a positive sign, but still it is difficult to stand by sometimes and watch you struggle, as, for example, when trying to find the brakes to your wheel chair with your uncooperative left hand.

Gity, Dr. Massoudi's assistant, came by to answer some questions. You can fly home. You will have from one to three titanium "plates" in your head (you actually ended up with four) to hold the flap in place, and these will not set off airport security (something I didn't ask). She will remind Dr. Massoudi that he has promised you a ride in his Ferrari. The last item, of course, is the most important. She said that given how well you are doing you shouldn't have any difficulty with the surgery, that usually the people who have problems are those who are quite ill when having the surgery. I hadn't thought of this. Also, she volunteered that you have been a very special patient to them, a "once in a blue moon" patient, someone who does far better than is expected.

Traci, from Rehab Without Walls, came this morning to do the assessment needed to begin planning your treatment back home. She was a bit surprised that you will be released so soon. She said that she would be writing up her assessment this afternoon. I'm so pleased this piece is now in place.

> *Memory (age 8, October): "It was raining and cold. You begged me to go outside and play catch. As stubborn as you are, I should have given in immediately instead of enduring your constant begging. I gave in. You were thrilled, and afterwards asked, happily, 'Aren't you glad you played.' Even though we were both a bit damp, I had to admit I was."*

October 24.

Dear Family and Friends,

In preparation for meeting Traci from Rehab Without Walls Adam wore a new T-shirt sent by Trent, a co-worker at the Children's Museum. The shirt read: "Pain Heals, Chicks Dig Scars, Glory Lasts Forever"

October 25th, Saturday, 10:28 a.m., California time.

Dear Adam:

You are having your speech therapy now, really cognitive therapy, which, ironically, seems mostly to involve work sheets (which you never liked as a kid). An example: the sheet you worked on Thursday required you to identify words—"very delicate"—that with the change of a single letter became something else—"part of a car" (Answer: And this took me some doing: "tender, fender." You quickly got some of these—a direction (east); changing the "t" to "y" you got the correct answer, "easy," something that is not challenging.

I've been trying to better understand how the damage to your mental machinery is influencing your thinking and action, and especially how you interact with others. When considered in relationship to the various stages of brain trauma recovery, which mostly illustrate how there really isn't a clear pattern to anything, that every person experiences much that is unique, I'm slowly beginning to understand a bit better some of what you are struggling with even as you are not really aware of the problems, at least not fully. The left hemisphere is the center of language, logic, time, and story, among other things. The right side of the brain attends to and lives in the moment, it is concerned with the constant flow of sensory stimuli, stuff that forms mental mosiacs, patchworks of images. It appears to make possible feelings of wonder and awe; some would say it's the place where God hangs out. But the majority of your damage is to the back of your head, where the cerebellum and occipital lobe are located. Damage to the cerebellum reaches across both sides of the brain.

In your behavior I see some elements of the patterns we have been told to look for. This said, it is the uniqueness of each injury that is most impressive, not the patterns. In any case, as I listen to you, and believe me, we all listen a lot, there is a matter-of-factness about how you see the world right now, things seem to fall into black and white, signs of an insistent moral dualism driven by a kind of grim facticity, a literalness to your experience. I better understand now why you got so frustrated when being teased just a bit; you took teasing as "playing with your head," and it's not funny. You are not very good at reading subtle cues given during speech and, as I've said before, you are very self-absorbed, and for good reason. When you are not the center of attention you quickly withdraw, sometimes then being quietly pouty and a bit punishing at least until the conversation turns back to you and your needs. You refuse to look at yourself in the mirror and while aware there is something called the future you are nearly overwhelmed by the present, the moment. The future enters your mind mostly (but not exclusively) in one way, getting home. In many respects, everything will get much, much, more difficult at home, especially for our family as we try to care for you.

You are very compliant toward requests made of you by your therapists, being almost childlike. Delightfully you chat with virtually everyone who comes by, which is a problem because you struggle with concentration. You really have difficulty walking and talking at the same time. When you talk, you have difficulty walking. Some of the therapeutic activities you turn into games, which makes sense since rules matter to you a lot.

When asked by Traci, the woman who assessed you yesterday, about whether or not you had walked stairs during therapy you said, "yes, there is a rule. Weak leg first when going down; strong leg first when going up." I think I've gotten the rule correct. You seem mostly unaware that others have struggles too, and that our lives have been dramatically changed by your injury—what matters is that you can't do what you formerly could do and that's unfair.

It's worth noting here that your speech patterns have an emphatic quality formerly lacking, a quality that is almost ministerial (in an Evangelical sense) in its confidence—and in wholly lacking humility. You speak as one who knows, while dismissing any possibility that others might reasonably disagree. Such people you dismiss as "idiots," a favorite word. (By the way, this morning when I said that Governor Sarah Palin isn't an idiot, she's bright but "just wrong on many issues" you said, "that's an idiot." You see what I mean, there is nothing subtle in how you are thinking right now— black, white.)

Cranioplasty: Trick, no Treat

October 26.

Dear Family and Friends,

Kirby stayed with Adam last night during which time he had a couple of nightmares, signaling, perhaps, a worried anticipation of tomorrow's cranioplasty. Strange dreams. In the first he is to stay in the hospital, saying that he must stay until he was able to do something with a bunch of letters spread out on his bed. He can't figure out what he is supposed to do, so he can't go home. In the second dream our family is standing around him while he was in bed. No one helps him but Kirby. He says, the "left side doesn't work, just cut it off."

12:40 p.m., California time. October 27.

Dear Adam:

I spent the night with you—about every 2 or so hours you needed to pee. Not much to show for the effort, but a need nonetheless. I didn't get much sleep. You were worried about surgery today, and you remain worried. Kirby came to your room an hour or so before your mother and Rachel. She began clearing stuff from the walls in anticipation of your move back to SICU after the surgery and your release from the hospital. She left for work and Rachel and your mom continued the work.

October 28.

Dear Family and Friends,

Adam's surgery went well last evening. He has a white turban tipping to the right and a single drain tube coming out of his head, one that ends in a bulb a bit like the end of a turkey baster but clear, that, when squeezed, provides just a bit of suction and slowly fills with blood mixed with brain fluid. Drainage is important to obtaining the desired internal pressure, otherwise a shunt once again becomes a possibility.

Adam spent last night in the SICU but because of two head trauma patients coming to the hospital in the last little while he has been moved to the Progressive Care Stroke Unit (PCSU) where he was before moving to Acute Rehab. He's in room 135—he started in room 16, moved to 14, then to 130, then 146, 102, 7, and now 135. Musical rooms.

The big event of the day: Just after a brief walker-assisted journey around the SICU and a bold attempt at eating lunch, Adam threw up.

Wednesday, October 29, 2:41 California time.

Dear Adam:

As I write, you are asleep. Your mother and I got to the hospital early this morning. Mom had been quite worried that you'd have had a rough night. We walked in and you seemed pretty chipper. You were chatting on the phone with Joshua who will fly in later tonight telling him that you were excited to see him.

Your mother and I need to pack Desmond this afternoon in anticipation of Joshua and me driving him home. You threw up three times yesterday and were a bit mean and very discouraged. You said you rested pretty well, had a dream about your head growing unevenly, but had an overall good night.

Dr. Chang came by and your mom gave him some cookies to say "thank you." He's become a special friend.

About 40 minutes ago Robert Ramirez who works as a volunteer in the SICU waiting room dropped by to take some pictures of our family and of him with us. He's a very kind man. You are very, very, tired. This surgery has really knocked you down. You haven't eaten much but you have peed.

The drain tube in your head with its attached clear rubber collector bulb has been miserable and we are waiting for Dr. Massoudi or Gity to come by and let us know if and when it can be removed. It drives you crazy. It looks to us that your head is draining very little now and the fluid is clearly getting less bloody. This said, we have no idea if this means the tube is ready to be removed. You are very anxious to get out of here, and we can't blame you. Earlier today a speech therapist dropped by to work with you. You answered all of her questions and demonstrated a pretty amazing memory, including remembering a set of words she told to you that you were supposed to keep in mind until asked. She told you the words, then you did about 10 minutes of work, and she asked you to repeat them. You did, without hesitation or a fault. She noted that you have some trouble concentrating which you dismissed as ADHD. I'd say having just had surgery might be a good explanation.

Finally, I should mention that you laugh about playing dumb as a strategy for manipulating your therapists. Not one of them, I think, is fooled. Quite the contrary.

Halloween. Friday, October 31.

Dear Family and Friends,

We've gotten the trick, not the treat... We'd hoped to bring Adam home today but, alas, his white count is still up, he has a slight cough, and he has an on-and-off fever which prevent his release. At 10:30 this morning he threw up what little breakfast he'd eaten. We fear Adam has an infection.

November 3.

Dear Family and Friends,

Fewer good signs today than yesterday—white count up, slight fever, vomited pizza (Little Caesar's...could it be the pizza?). Adam is now in room 143, moved there because of a difficult new young roommate. Dawn Ann and Rachel have struggled all day to get Adam to eat, sit up, even talk. It took considerable convincing to get him to talk on the phone with his Grandfather Bullough, who Adam believes understands his struggles as others do not because of having had a battle with his health a year ago himself. At one point Adam said that he wasn't going to talk to anyone until he is home. Fortunately, he promised to phone his grandpa, and he did. Adam keeps his promises.

November 6.

Dear Family and Friends,

Adam has had yet another setback. We know that the infection is Enterobacter, the same infection that afflicted his lungs in September. He will have surgery tomorrow to determine the extent of the infection and whether or not the bone flap needs to be removed.

> *Medical memo: "Risk factors for nosocomial Enterobacter infections include hospitalization of greater than 2 weeks, invasive procedures in the past 72 hours, treatment with antibiotics in the past 30 days, and the presence of a central venous catheter... Enterobacter species can cause disease in virtually any body compartment."* [12]

"If I die..."

Today is Day 87. November 7. 5:45 p.m. California time.

Dear Adam:

We are waiting to see you. You are in post op and will be brought shortly to SICU and put into isolation. Isolation means we get to wear yellow paper gowns and gloves. I flew in last night to Long Beach—a less expensive flight and a better time for getting to see you for a little while before going to Heidi's house. Mom and I made the decision for me to fly to California at the last minute only after finding out that you would be having surgery today. No time was given. I thought about driving so we'd have a car and I could bring some of your's and your sister's stuff with me that Joshua and I brought home but with the possibility that surgery would be done early I gave up on this idea.

The last few days have been very, very difficult. Your mother and I have been on the phone a lot. She's been in tears. I've worried but haven't felt you were in danger. Mostly my concern has been for your spirits, a concern that has prominently weighed on your mother. On the way from the airport to the hospital your mom said that you were looking forward to seeing me. When I arrived we spoke a little, but you gave no sign of being all that pleased by my arrival. But, I knew you were: You had kept yourself awake to see me even though you were exhausted. You have been frightened. In fact, your mother reports that yesterday afternoon teary-eyed you told her you were "scared" and then said, "If I die I'll say 'hi' to Grandma [Mortensen]." I got you talking some today and while the mood wasn't light you did laugh when we read to you the statements on the Chuck Norris t-shirt Kirby bought you ("Chuck Norris refers to himself in fourth person"). You were worried, and your fears were heightened by waiting...and waiting.

I should mention that Dr. Sarafian, an infectious disease specialist, came by this morning and looked at your head. Although your mother mentioned to me on the phone a couple of days ago that you had a wound near your right temple that was draining, I couldn't quite visualize it. I got only a brief glance today and it is worrisome.

Surgery was scheduled for 2 p.m. You were supposed to leave your room at 1:30 but 1:30 came and went, then 2:00...finally you were on your way at 3:20. You went straight to the operating room where you were prepped. Wearing yellow isolation robes and surgical gloves we said a family prayer late this morning. (I took off my gloves to hold your hand.) Before leaving for surgery I gave you a blessing, promising you that the bone flap would not need to be removed and that the surgery would be short and go well. I must say that after I said these things I worried. Happily, you and we were blessed on each count.

The four of us, Kirby, Rachel, your mother and I have agreed that we will not tell you what Dr. Massoudi just said about leaving the hospital (reported below). We do not want to get your hopes up. A positive surprise is what we hope for. If everything goes well, you'll most certainly be here for about another week. At home you'll continue to have nuclear antibiotics, an IV. Dr. Massoudi said that the decision not to remove your bone flap made sense, but you will be closely monitored. There is still a possibility that it will die and begin to be reabsorbed into your body. If this happens, we are looking at another surgery then perhaps six months of wearing a helmet—but you'd be home—and then returning here to have reconstructive surgery. I have a feeling this won't be necessary.

As you were wheeled into the operating room and we said our "good byes," I said to you, "not to worry, everything will go all right." In a flat voice, you said, "I hope so." As I write we are waiting to see you. Soon you will be back in SICU where so many love you. You will be in isolation. Your mom has said many times that she wonders why we are still in California. She worries about many things in addition to your health and well-being, including running out of sick leave days at work. I spent much of yesterday trying to sort out insurance issues and made little progress. (I'm tempted to say to everyone, "Adam's taken out bankruptcy, too bad....") I'm not certain there are reasons for many things in life, but this I know: We have a choice about how we respond to the challenges we face. We are learning and growing as a family, getting stronger and I think better. But it's sure not easy.

November 7.

Dear Family and Friends,

Adam just came out of surgery. While we were in the SICU waiting room, a place that is all too familiar to us, Dr. Massoudi came and shared the following information: The bone flap looked good although there was a good deal of infection—mushy stuff—that needed to be cleaned out and flushed. The brain is not involved. Adam had a place on the right side of his forehead that looked like a small scab that oozed. This was repaired. Two drains were inserted, one high and one low on the wound. If everything goes well—Dr. Massoudi gave odds of 2 out of 3—Adam will be in SICU through the weekend and in the hospital through next week and then be able to come home where he will be on IV antibiotics.

Hope

November 9.

Dear Family and Friends,

Early this morning Seth flew into Long Beach from Salt Lake. We didn't tell Adam he was coming; actually we didn't know until late last night. Arriving at the hospital, Seth quickly donned the yellow uniform and wandered into Room 8. Looking up and seeing his brother, actually two Seths—one of the benefits of double vision—Adam began crying and they embraced. Soon the brothers were happily chatting, laughing, and enjoying one another's company. Dawn Ann cried as well. A beautiful moment.

9:42 a.m., November 10. Monday.

Dear Adam:

I just left your room. Seth, Rachel, and your mother are still there. I know you are nervous and anxious but right now it's hard for me to listen to you. You are eating very little. You don't "like" the cereal, you say (so why order it?). At this point, liking what you eat seems to me irrelevant. You are lying in bed and you have done little to keep up on the breathing exercises you are supposed to do to avoid getting pneumonia. Discouraging.

Mom and I have been very worried about what is ahead. I simply don't know how I am going to find the time, energy, and ability to sort through the insurance, Social Security and Medicaid issues. I don't even know where to begin. I spent a day last week trying to make sense of some of the insurance problems, made lots of phone calls, but didn't get much help or direction.

My mother's advice was probably best—"Don't pay anything, wait." Unfortunately, I paid three bills last Thursday before flying to California. Technically and legally, I believe we aren't responsible for any of this, but here we are.

We are waiting to hear the results of the CAT scan. Also, we don't know anything about the blood clot in your right arm—size, position, threat. Hopefully your head has healed enough for you to be given a blood thinner. Because of the clot the PICC line was put in your left arm, which I'd guess will interfere with your rehab. I don't know why another place wasn't selected. Nuts.

Kirby is getting ill. A cold, I think.

You said that your temperature was "low" through the night, which is very good, perhaps indicating that the drugs are knocking down the infection. So, lots to be grateful for.

I leave tomorrow morning for home. Seth leaves Wednesday. Rachel and your mother will then be on their own. Hopefully we'll have a date for your departure which will make everything else flow much more smoothly. Much still needs to be done in Salt Lake.

An addition: It is now 2:16 p.m., same day. At 10:30 I returned from writing the above and after sitting down I asked, "Any word on the white count." Your mother quickly shushed me. You've gone from a 12 to a 15, the wrong direction. My heart sank at the news and a quick feeling of panic and despair hit me. When everyone left for a moment you said to me, "Dad, I'm losing hope, I'll never get out of here." Shortly thereafter I checked with your nurse who looked up your scores. No temp. Kidneys normal. We really do not know what the raise in white count means.

Your mother, Seth and Rachel just returned from Yogurtland. While they were gone Maria, one of the nurses' aides, came by. She brings such happiness with her. I am so grateful to her; she lightens your burdens. On your part, you point out that she is very, very funny, but since I don't speak Spanish I'll never know. "She's a happy person," you said. While I was in the bathroom the phone rang. Billie from the insurance company. Saying she is overwhelmed by our bills she has made arrangements for us to have a person to serve as a sort of bill manager, an accountant, to work with us; Billie will continue as case manager. This is a relief. We need help.

November 11.

Dear Family and Friends,

Adam has been very down. He won't look at anyone who comes to see him. Grace, the nurse's assistant, was so saddened to see him this way, remembering when he would talk and talk and make her laugh, that she bought him at the hospital gift shop a cross with the word LOVE on it.

November 12, 10:25 Utah time.

Dear Adam:

I am in Salt Lake. Shortly after walking into the house the phone rang. Rachel said that Dr. Massoudi had visited and told you that you would be home in two or three days. I was stunned. Earlier your mother said the white count had only dropped slightly, from 15 something to 14.6. A flurry of phone calls followed and I began scrambling. I had spoken with Billie who promised to give me a list of physicians. We agreed I would call when I arrived home, which I did. I got the list, some of whom turned out to be specialists in such things as AIDS, and started working. I'm so glad that already I had made arrangements for a rehab physician and Rehab Without Walls. Now, we need to get an infectious disease specialist and a neurosurgeon. I think things are now arranged, or shortly will be arranged, for you to work with physicians at the University of Utah. I have an appointment set for a week from this coming Friday. (Here I should mention that your bug is Enterobacter, the same bug you've had all along, and that the drug you are being given every eight hours is 2000 mg of Meurpinem.) I also spoke with the people at the University's neurosurgery clinic and, after having described what amounts to a very complicated process for getting you transferred, I asked if everything could be expedited if Dr. Massoudi's office would call. I was told this would move things along. Unfortunately, I couldn't get anyone at Dr. Massoudi's office nor at Dr. Sarafian's, so I left detailed messages. The problem is that a physician needs to make these referrals.

There's No Place Like Home

Friday, November 14, 4:07 p.m., Utah time. Day 94.

Dear Adam:

It's been a crazy day. Your mother and I have been working to get everything in place for you to return home. I've made flight arrangements so that you, Rachel, and your mother arrive today on a Delta flight at 3:43 p.m. There has been a lot to get done and not everything is in place. For instance, this morning Shelly at Dr. Massoudi's office told me that she can't set things up with a neurosurgeon here which I had been told could be done by a person at the clinic at the University. The case manager at Mission Hospital, I find out, is supposed to do these things. I wish someone had told us this. I started phoning people early this morning, sometime around 5 a.m. and leaving messages. The first was to Billie at the insurance company to get authorizations. I really do not know how many calls I've made. I just got off the phone with Billie a few minutes ago; she confirmed authorization has been given for Rehab Without Walls—which begins tomorrow morning, something you won't like followed by another session at 1 p.m. She's also authorized a wheel chair and walker. A raised toilet is not covered by insurance but Grandpa Mortensen has one of these from when Grandma was ill. Today I also built a small ramp for the back door and again raked the lawns and the side of the house so wheeling you to the back door won't be too difficult or messy. I also cut the front lawn. Now, lots to do inside.

I can only imagine how excited you must be. Now, the really hard work begins. Yesterday afternoon when we got news that your white count had risen to 15 my heart sank. I went on line and looked up white count measures, phoned your mother, and read her some of the information. (I should note that today she didn't check the numbers, saying she "didn't want to know." She used Dr. Chang's sense of where you are to justify her action, noting that it isn't necessary to be tested every day, that the antibiotics need time to do their work, and the numbers aren't very helpful anyway.)

Over the past several weeks most of the folks who visited you in the first several weeks faded. Life really does have to go on—but ours hasn't. I'm so glad for your mother and Rachel who need badly to be home. This said, for Rachel returning comes with mixed feelings. I think she loves Matt.

November 14.

Dear Family and Friends,

Dawn Ann, Rachel and Kirby went to the hospital at 9 a.m. and found Adam with eyes closed and resting. There was a knot in Dawn Ann's stomach. She was sure that someone would say that Adam could not go home today because of something...

Before getting on the plane Adam was frisked and checked carefully, including wheel chair and eye patch, just in case he is a terrorist who cannot hold up his head let alone walk or run. He was put on the plane before anyone else and allowed to use the bathroom before the flight began. Because of maintenance problems, the flight was delayed 30 minutes. Arriving in Salt Lake City Adam was exhausted but happy. Bob Patio, Uncle Richard, cousin Garrett, Grandma and Grandpa Bullough waited anxiously in the airport, checking and rechecking arrival times and positioning themselves so when Adam, Rachel, and Dawn Ann deplaned they could not be missed. Last to leave the airplane, a joyous reunion followed. Hurrying home a nurse met us and Adam was hooked up to an IV. Vorn had decorated the house with balloons and a large "WELCOME HOME, ADAM" banner and lots of family and several friends gathered to celebrate Adam's return. He ate our friend Corina's pizza then crashed.

November 15.

Dear Family and Friends,

Quite a day. Bob slept downstairs in the guest bedroom. Dawn Ann slept in our bedroom which is now Adam's bedroom. Neither one of us got much sleep. Rachel slept with her dog...upstairs. We have learned a lot in one day; in many respects we are beginning a new day count, a new journey. The constants are lots of peeing, lots of sleeping, struggling over eating, some socially inappropriate behavior and complaining, lots of medical people coming in and out of our lives but with different faces than those we came to love at Mission Hospital, tons of paperwork, and, of course, skinny, boney, little Adam.

Layla, the dog, is replacing the neuropsychologist at Mission Hospital who advised us on Adam but didn't meet with him—she simply assumed he was a member of a class, a category, "brain injured young men." Layla, in contrast, has better credentials, including furriness, a wet nose, and a great deal of interest in Adam—and an firmer pawshake.

Needles, Therapy, and a Sucky Life

Dear Adam:

As I write, you are meeting with Maren, a speech therapist. Earlier today Heather, an occupational therapist, met with you. Heather seemed willing to have you more or less set the limits of what you do. I told her, out of your hearing, that you are very compliant when a therapist asks you to do something and that she shouldn't hesitate to push you, that you are quite contented to limit your work. I know, not nice.

Last night was my night to stay with you. Both your mother and Rachel have had their turns, and both have chosen to sleep with you which I cannot do. I have enough difficulty sleeping. Out of kindness your mother set up the inflatable mattress for me at the foot of your (our) bed. It's horrible. It's short, noisy, squishy, and, well, simply impossible for a body like mine. Last night around 10 o'clock I hooked you up to the IV while your mother went to bed downstairs in the guest bedroom. At 11:45 the IV was finished, much slower than the package reads (15-30 minutes). You peed only twice during the night, using the pee bottles which I only had to empty once. At 5 something I got up and checked my email while waiting to begin your 6 a.m. IV. I was doing this when your mom came up stairs. I then went downstairs and read for a while and fell asleep, sleeping until nearly 9 a.m. when your therapist arrived.

As the days since Friday have passed, we are getting a pretty good idea of what we are facing. Last night you had a bit of a temperature, which really got me worrying (and no doubt worried you—several times you stuck a thermometer in your mouth and took your temperature). Your body remains a biological battle ground. The white medical cap you wear has marks on it from your wounds draining. (Oh, by the way, while we were at church yesterday, you took a shower. Wonderful! Your mom seemed very pleased. Seth helped you. Thank goodness for Seth!)

Just before the therapist arrived this afternoon your mother returned from spending the morning at Wasatch Elementary School. She said she cried as she approached the school. She's been away from work a long time. She's hoping to spend some time over the next few days at the school learning about her duties from the substitute librarians before taking over.

Lots to do. I'm waiting to hear from the University about a neurosurgeon. The goal is to have the flap staples out by the 24th of November. My mother called about visiting you and so did Grandpa Mortensen. You gave your mother grief yesterday for letting some people visit who stayed overly long, exhausting you. These visits prevented a couple of your friends from visiting. You said that your mom "didn't think it through." Truth is, we're just beginning to learn how to handle visitors—last night you told us to tell Corina and Richardo Ayala that they could visit but that you couldn't "handle children." They said they'd visit another time. Most folks, like your grandparents and the Ayalas, are very sensitive to the situation and everyone is understanding.

November 18.

Dear Family and Friends,

Being home is so very nice.

Adam's morning begins with a 6:00 a.m. infusion of IV antibiotics. We let him sleep while we hook him up to the IV, and an hour later he is done, and still sleeping. Then we battle with trying to get him to wake up around 8:00 a.m. His therapy sessions begin around 9:00 a.m., so we want him up, dressed and breakfast done. Most mornings he does well although today he ate breakfast while the speech therapist worked with him. She actually was glad to have him eating so she can see how he is doing swallowing. Antibiotic infusions also are at 2 and 10 p.m.

The great news is that he slept in the room alone last night.

November 20, 9:58 a.m., Utah time.

Dear Adam:

I just helped you walk, with your cane, into the east bathroom. While you were getting dressed I said, "You look great, Adam." "No I don't, I won't look good until I am normal and can play the guitar. My life sucks." No doubt this is true, but from where we have been, trust me, you look great and you have a life. For this we shall always be grateful. Returning from the bathroom (which is quite a complex operation of measuring each step), at the base of the stairs you found Layla blocking your way. "Move, Layla." She didn't get up in response to your command, but she shifted, slightly. You then very carefully and patiently stepped over her tail with the support of your cane first getting your less-than-obedient left leg up and over followed by your stronger and more obedient right leg. Having successfully maneuvered around Layla, you worked your way towards the bed.

Dr. Sarafian phoned and spoke with your mom yesterday. He was kindly checking on how you are doing and was encouraging, suggesting that some additional tests of how your infection is responding to the antibiotics—he calls them "antibeeotics"—suggest that soon you can be put on a once a day dosage. This would be wonderful. When your mother told me this, I said, "All I care about is that the infection is eradicated, that it doesn't return."

I just helped you get to the computer where you are downloading some pictures Kirby sent. As you downloaded a picture I began replacing the light switch in the dining room. Suddenly you called to me to come and help you get to bed. You were very upset. Somehow you saw some pictures of yourself, of your stomach surgery. "I'm a mess," you said, as we shuffled into the bedroom. I can't blame you. Truth is, you aren't yet fully aware of how you look nor, really, of what you have gone through. Knowledge of this kind must await another day and time, some time in the future after you are more of who you once were....

November 22, day 102.

Dear Adam:

After peeing, you crawled into the utility room and are sitting at the computer. Getting around Layla, who is quite content to stay put and be in the way, again proved difficult. When you are finished we will go upstairs where you'll ride the recumbent bike. Yesterday I didn't get your meds started until 2:30 so when Lisa arrived at 3 p.m. you had a good excuse for not going upstairs and riding. Instead, you stayed downstairs and she had you work with weights and with the stretchy straps that provide a bit of resistance to build muscle strength as you pull them. Later, however, she got you upstairs. How, I do not know. You rode the bike for about ten minutes and enjoyed it, saying later that you could feel your muscles working. I'm delighted. You said that I needed to take you upstairs and explain how the machine is programmed. Glad to do it.

Since it's Saturday, no therapy today, which is all right with you even though at some level you must know that not working isn't helping you get better. Still, I suspect your body needs periodic breaks and so perhaps this is a good use of time. As I write, Rachel and your mother are out somewhere returning dishes to people who kindly have provided meals this past week and picking up things, including gift certificates, for people who helped with the house and animals while we were away.

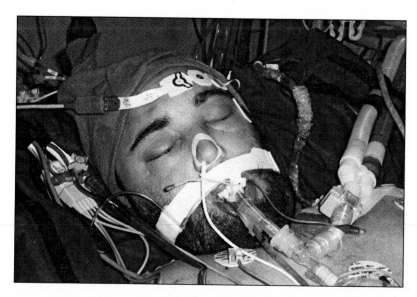

Coma

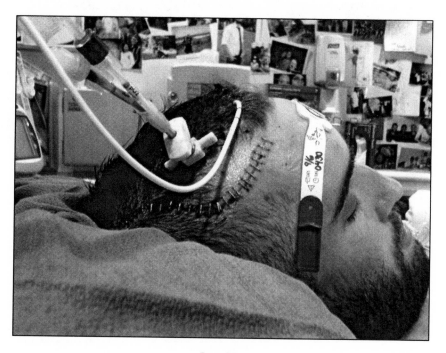

Day 25

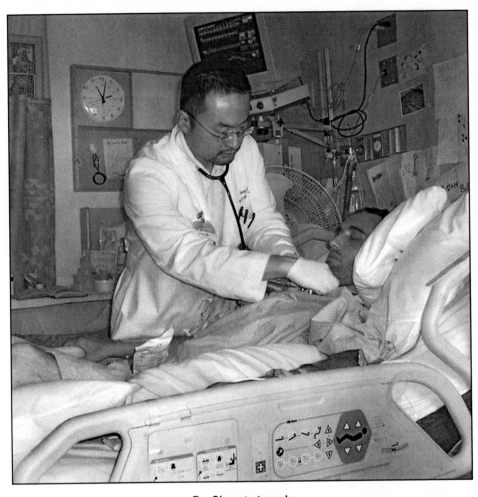

Dr. Chang at work

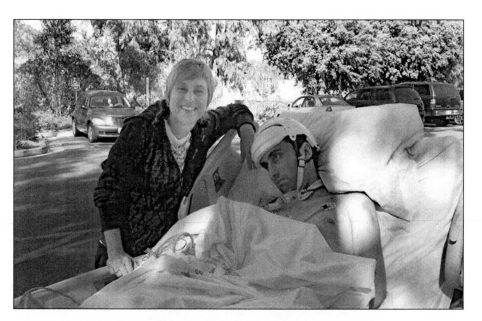

Going outside for the first time

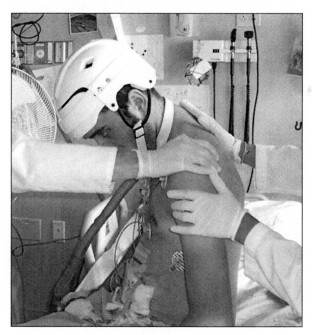

Sitting up

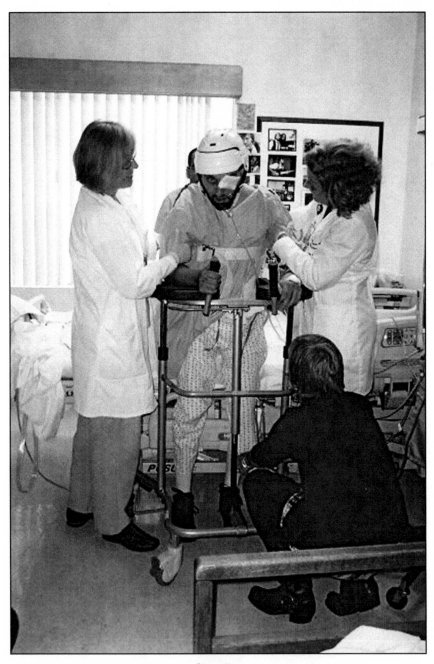

Standing

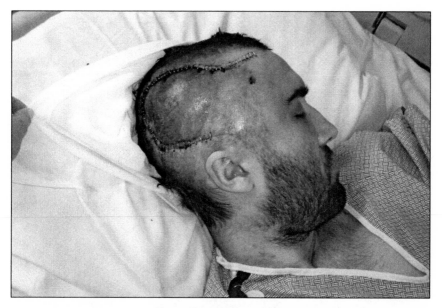

Bone flap replacement

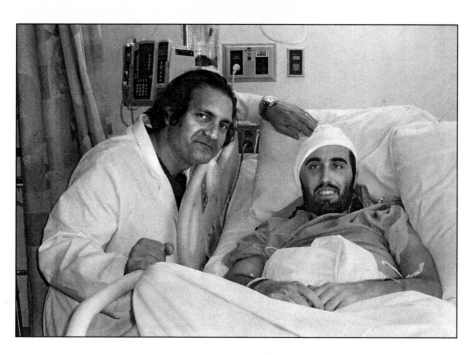

Dr. Massoudi and Adam

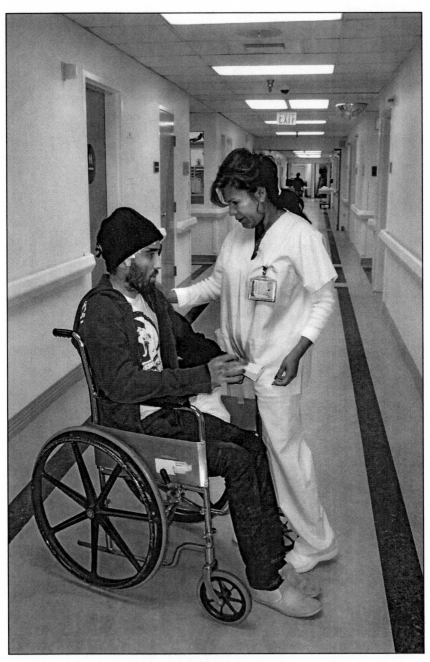

Saying "goodbye" to Maria

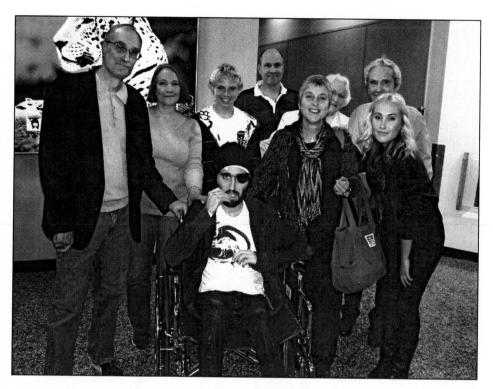

Airport homecoming

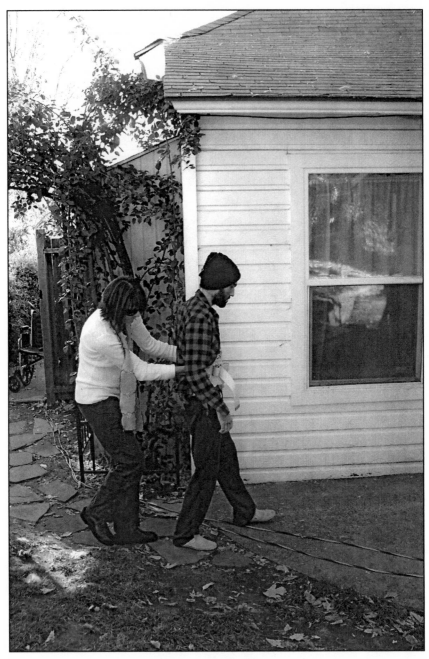

Walking home with Lisa

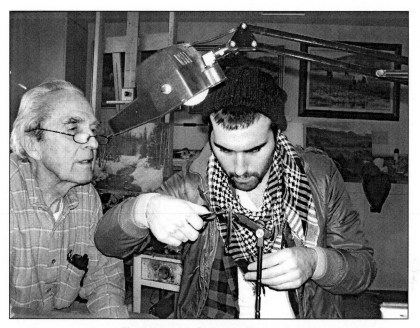

Fly tying with Grandpa Bullough

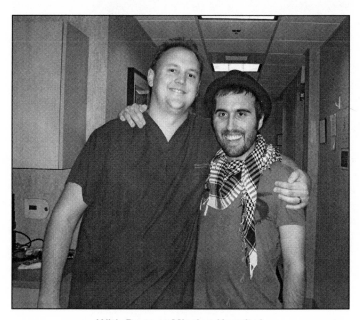

With Dave at Mission Hospital

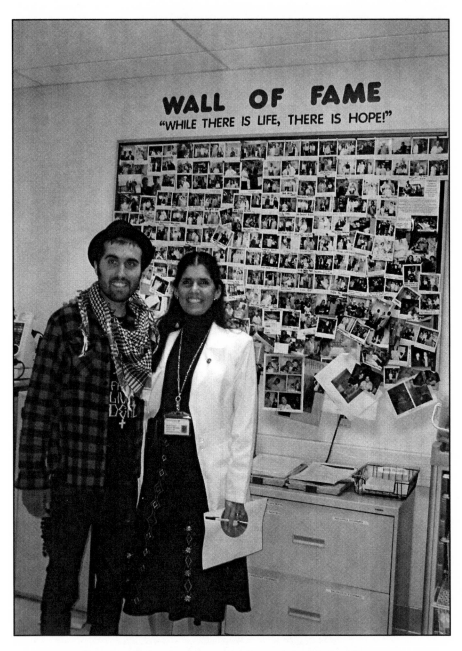

Mary Kay Bader and Adam in front of the Wall of Fame

Head Staples and Giving Thanks

Monday, November 24.

Dear Adam:

This morning we took you to University Hospital for an appointment in the hope that your staples would be removed. When Melody, who works with Dr. Jensen, the neurosurgeon, saw your head, she asked if it had been covered and what had been done. She seemed just a bit surprised that you still had a bandage and were wearing a cap. When I first saw your wound, which was covered in bloody goo and seemed to me to look pretty bad, I wondered what was going on. It turns out that according to her, although she didn't say this directly, that despite what your mother was told to do by the PCSU nurses at Mission Hospital, your head should have been exposed to the air and allowed to dry and heal. She said that moisture of this sort coupled with darkness is just what bacteria need to grow. Made sense. While she tried to avoid being critical of what was done, it was clear she wasn't pleased as indicated by her statement that another couple of weeks of antibiotics is a good idea. When she first uncovered your head and after looking at it for a moment, originally thinking, I believe, that she would have a relatively easy time deciding whether or not to remove the staples (it turns out there are also some sutures), she got a resident to look at you. Looking and then picking away at some of the stuff, he concluded we need to wait for another week. So, Monday we'll go in again and this time we hope all the staples will be removed (some were today—which I asked Melody to do if possible). Your mother obviously felt very badly about the situation, saying three times that she only did what she was told, and she did, faithfully.

You were very disappointed about not getting all the staples removed today. On the way to the car you stopped before getting into the front seat. I didn't understand what you were doing. You told me that you were looking at your "reflection," which I then noticed. You are quite concerned about how you look and worry about what Kirby will think when she arrives Thursday morning.

November 27, Thanksgiving day. It is 7:18 p.m., Utah time.

Dear Adam:

Your mother has pulled off an amazing event. Somewhere around 37 people have been here for Thanksgiving dinner. Dessert is just about finished. You are sitting on your bed (our, your mother's and my, bed), Kirby is sitting on your right, and you are eating a piece of your mother's pumpkin pie. She made the pie last night. I helped peel and cut up the pumpkins but the magic is all hers. I picked up Kirby, Emmely and Heidi at the airport this morning shortly before 11 a.m. Heidi loves people, and I think she's had a good day and evening. Kirby has been terrific with you. It was fun for me to go in and out of the bedroom to and from the Study and hear the two of you chatting, mostly you talking, and cuddling a bit. Your head still looks pretty gruesome, but she doesn't seem to mind.

The sleeping plan is for Kirby to have your room downstairs and for Emmely and Heidi to share the guest bedroom. Your mother will sleep on the inflatable camping bed and I'll be in the Study.

Yesterday we took you to see Dr. Jensen. Melody and Dr. Jensen removed the last of the stitches and staples, which was something your mother had prayed would happen. You seemed pleased. This morning you took a shower and washed your head, something that was badly needed. Last night Seth trimmed your hair and beard. You were getting ready for Kirby and wanted to look your best today. You don't seem overly self-conscious about your wounds, which is terrific. Dr. Jensen said something that was very interesting. After being told about what the nurses in Mission Hospital had told you and your mother about caring for your head, he said they were treating a "head wound like any other wound" but the head is different, more delicate and much more serious.

November 28.

Dear Family and Friends,

Kirby made a comment today that really sums up many of my feelings—She said, "It's been two weeks since I last saw you, and LOOK AT YOU!" He had just walked, slowly and deliberately with hand tightly gripping the rail, down stairs—he and Kirby had watched a movie (because of his double vision, Adam wore an eye patch on the outside of his glasses)—to the main floor of the house.

November 28.

Dear Adam:

We spoke with Mark, the Rehab Without Walls social worker, today after he finished his session with you. We asked about your view of your situation, noting that you seem to believe that your brain is just fine, that the challenge before you is to regain your coordination and strength. Your mother mentioned, and Kirby confirmed that you made a similar comment to her, that you should be all right in about three weeks. Oh, if it were only so! Three weeks!

On his last visit I asked Mark to check into Medicaid and Social Security, which I've let drop. He did so, saying that Medicaid is probably out but that we should apply for Social Security. We will, he said—and others have said the same thing—be turned down but you should qualify. You seem a bit concerned about your finances, a topic that your mother brought up with Mark asking how we should handle the situation. You are running through what little money you have rather quickly. The advice we were given was to think of you like an adolescent. (Now, where did we hear this before? Oh, yeah, that helpful neuropsychologist at Mission Hospital!) I know this will trouble you because you most certainly do not think of yourself in this way, but it may be good advice. He said a similar thing when we discussed the challenge of helping you come to terms with being brain-injured and not just physically hurt. On my and your mother's part, we simply pray for your complete recovery.

You've done a lot of crawling around today. Watching you crawl upsets me even as I recognize that crawling indicates a growing independence and, as you've pointed out, it strengthens your arms. Here I should mention that I went upstairs with you and while holding the rail you moved fairly quickly and well until getting to the top where it's difficult to find places to hold on. I watched you from the dinner table crawling toward the bathroom with Kirby tagging along behind. As so often happens, Layla was in your way and she had no intention of moving. Earlier, at the table, Layla came into the dining room; your mother urged her to leave. This led to a funny interaction about Layla, that she really thinks she is a person even though in the pre-existence she raised her hands to volunteer to be a dog. You didn't think this was funny.

I hate to see you suffer.

> *Memory (age nine, May): "You had a wonderful birthday. You were very excited—money has a way of doing this to you. As the doorbell rang, you rushed to answer proclaiming, 'Another customer!' The bad news is that you got lots of money which signaled the beginning of your harassment of your mother and me. 'Mom,' you said, 'can we go to Toys R Us?' You see, you can't stand to have money without spending it. Right this minute my desk drawer is filled with Watermelon Jolly Rancher candies. When I found them and asked where they came from you said, 'I only bought five dollars worth.'"*

On Food...and Family

December 1.

Dear Family and Friends,

After doing the early morning infusion today, Dawn Ann returned to work at Wasatch Elementary School. The principal, Julie Miller, the faculty and children, have been wonderfully supportive of Dawn Ann and Adam, so Dawn Ann was excited to return. As I write, she's in bed after a very long day, exhausted. Among the high points of the day for Dawn Ann was having a child insist on leaving money with her to replace a lost book but not knowing the book title, cost, or even if it is, in fact, lost.

December 2.

Dear Family and Friends,

Dawn Ann reports that the children at school ask about Adam. They want to know when he will be coming back. They want him back to teach P.E. The children don't really fully understand the extent of Adam's injury. It surprises them to learn that he is learning to walk again and that he will not be back to teach them this year.

December 2. 11:35 a.m.

Dear Adam:

As I write you have just begun your therapy session with Heather. Earlier this morning you showered. We all run around trying to help you. We worry you might slip. So, I check on you frequently, the last time you said that you were "almost ready." I returned to the computer where I was working. Shortly after sitting down I could hear you calling, "Dad, DAD, DAD!" Frustrated, I shouted, "Wait a minute!" Walking into the bathroom, you said, "When I told you I was almost ready I meant I was almost ready." Apparently you expected me to stand outside of the shower and wait. Even while you are becoming increasingly independent, caring for you is exhausting.

Having returned to work on Monday your mom's routine of old is in place with some twists. She gets up about 4:30 a.m. and rides the recumbent bike. Around 6 a.m. she begins your infusion of antibiotics, showers and gets ready for school and cooks you breakfast. This morning you awakened long after she had left for school so your Popeye eggie breakfast was waiting, cold. Rachel brought it to you. Like so many other mornings you complained that your mother hadn't cooked the egg correctly, that there wasn't any yoke for you to dip your bread. I offered to cook you another egg but you refused, saying you weren't hungry after having finished the high calorie Carnation drink she made for you. While in coma, you lost a lot of weight.

It is now 1:40 p.m. Your therapist just left and you are in the bathroom. I went to the grocery store and got stuff to make you a sandwich which I made a few minutes ago. What was your response?: "You made it too thick, I can't open my mouth that wide." I gave it to Rachel and made you another, thinner, sandwich, not saying a word.

Still December 2nd but now 2:30. You've eaten the entire sandwich and called to me, "Dad, Dad... That was a really good sandwich." I needed that, thank you. Love, Dad.

Christmas, 2008, part of a Letter to Our Friends:

Dear Friends,

What a year! As a child, I recall being asked to write on the first day of school a brief piece on "How I spent my summer vacation." Since it is difficult to recall anything of 2008 before this summer, I'll begin with our summer vacation and then reach backwards for a story or two. In early June, our dear friend and my mentor, Paul Klohr, died. We were unable to attend the memorial service held for Paul at his home in Columbus because Dawn Ann's mother's health suddenly deteriorated and she passed away on the 10th of July. Happily, Adam, who was living in California and seeking work, was able to fly home to attend his grandmother's funeral which, as far as funerals go, was a celebration of a life very well lived. While we were grateful that Annetta would no longer face a future of prolonged suffering, we feel her absence constantly. So, June and July were bad months. Surely, August would be better.

The evening of Tuesday, August 12th, after Bob returned home from his bishopric meeting we received a phone call from Adam's girlfriend, Kirby. Hearing Kirby's voice, Dawn Ann immediately knew something was seriously wrong. Adam, Kirby said, had been hurt in a fall off his bicycle. More phone calls followed and as Adam underwent surgery Dawn Ann and I tried to find a flight to Orange County. There were none. The next morning we were met at the Long Beach Airport by Kirby's mom, Heidi, and a family friend, Jay Mortensen, who drove us to Mission Hospital in Mission Viejo, California. Adam's injury was worse than anything we could have imagined. Traumatic brain injury... Many weeks in a coma. Infections. Acute Respiratory Distress. Days of wondering if Adam would live or die piled on top of one another and blended into a deepening exhaustion and lingering fear, and then, following a terrible trial of faith, there came a remarkable miracle that still unfolds. Many, perhaps most of you, have followed on the Caringbridge web page the journey we have been on since Adam's fall so I will not repeat what is written there. Except for one visit home for Dawn Ann and trips back and forth so I could teach my Wednesday night class and attend as best as I could to my ecclesiastical and other responsibilities, from August 13th to mid November we lived in California with Heidi's family. Rachel dropped her classes for fall term, quit her job, and joined us about a week after Adam fell. During this time we have been the recipients of countless acts of kindness, have made new and unexpected friendships, have witnessed superhuman efforts made by nurses and physicians on Adam's behalf, and have been given a glimpse into goodness, make that a capital G (Goodness), that has been renewing, humbling, and a clear manifestation of grace. As a family, we think we have grown, and for this too we are grateful.

So, that's how we spent our summer vacation.

Merry Christmas and God bless, the Bulloughs.

December 6, 9:30 p.m. Day 116.

Dear Adam:

It's almost 9:30 p.m., Sunday. Your mother and I have been upstairs watching a Hallmark presentation, a story about a young man with Tourette's Syndrome who wanted to be a teacher. A beautiful story. You, Rachel and a few friends have been downstairs watching the latest Batman movie. You've been in a good mood and quite funny. While watching TV your mother suddenly began crying, and not because of the story. I asked her what was wrong. "Oh, nothing," she said. But when I pressed a bit for an answer she said, "It's everything, Adam, my mother's death."

At dinner tonight you told a story of having members of the Crips gang live in your building while you served your mission. You said that they kind of befriended you after you took out the garbage a few times for them. They showed you a hand shake, and apparently called out to you, "Hey, Adam," when seeing you, and gave you gang signs and sometimes shook your hand—it's a shake that involves bumping fists and snapping fingers. In any case, I made a comment that it seems to me that you went too far when you had the scar on your head shaped into a C. You laughed, and said that "Massoudi probably tried to put a Z but didn't have room." You were really funny. This was the first time you have actually come to the dining room table sat and eaten with us. Joshua, Vorn, Seth, Rachel, and the two young cousins were present. You didn't like the ham, so after you ate some salad I heated up some of the stew I made the other evening and you ate that. You said that your taste isn't yet "normal." I must say, finding things you will eat is a big part of our lives. You are demanding but mostly appreciative.

December 8.

Dear Adam:

It's a bit after 8 o'clock, p.m. I just walked through our (your) bedroom on the way to the Study and overheard you say to Kirby over the phone, "I pissed standing up." I stopped, and said, "That's not appropriate." "It's progress, Dad," you retorted. Okay.

December 9. Day 119.

Dear Family and Friends,

Adam has difficulty multitasking. He's easily distracted and has to work to stay focused. After helping in the school library, Dawn Ann spoke with him about how to talk with the children, reminding him of the importance of looking at them, making eye contact, and paying attention. As Lisa, his therapist, pointed out, having to shelve books was a good cognitive exercise for Adam, and she's right. He thought it boring, but clearly enjoyed being in the library.

December 13. Saturday.

Dear Family and Friends,

Ah, what a day—No more PICC line, all 36 cm gone with a tug; no more little invaders, presumably all deservedly dead; no more early morning infusions, and the seemingly endless drip, drip, and drip of Ertapenem; no more showers taken left arm protected by a plastic bag held in place by two rubber bands, one arm pit high the other elbow low; and no more PolarPack Temperature Assurance Material-protected drugs, "Discard after December 14." A very good day, and a step toward greater independence. Tomorrow is one month to the day of Adam's homecoming. Merry Christmas. (We have some wonderful stocking stuffers and we are willing to share: Let's see, we have 29 09% sodium chloride injection syringes; 11 Heparin Lock Flush Solution syringes; 7 Rate Flow Regulator IV sets, 4 Dressing Change Kits, 1 Diphenhydramine syringe I—use for severe drug-induced allergic reaction, good until May 27th—1 Epinephrine with a filtered needle, also good to May 27th, and a box of medium VersaPro lightly powdered latex exam gloves. The gloves have several interesting potential uses most of which are probably legal.)

Normal?

Dear Adam:

I should mention that Thursday morning we met with Dr. Ryser. Lisa, one of your Rehab Without Walls therapists who has been wonderful with you, attended the meeting, and it's a good thing she did. The paperwork we thought had been sent to Dr. Ryser from California apparently has been either lost or not sent. I screwed up by misunderstanding your mother's directions and bringing the wrong folder of materials to the meeting. Part of the meeting, a small part, involved us telling him about the changes in you we've noticed. I told the truth, as I see it, which made me and you a bit uncomfortable but I do not think anyone is well served by ignoring things. Wanting desperately to be seen as normal, you put a positive spin on everything and argue that you really haven't changed at all. After I said what I thought I needed to say, and you were clearly not happy about it, Dr. Ryser made an effort to get you to understand that what I said really has nothing to do with you and everything to do with brain injury, that he saw in my comments the typical patterns of TBI. I am concerned that if we suggest that everything is dandy a decision will be made to limit your therapy, and that would be a disaster. The longer we can prolong Rehab Without Walls the better, I think. Near the end of the meeting, Dr. Ryser suggested that a thorough analysis of how you are doing by a neuropsychologist would be helpful to planning your therapy, so we are in the process of figuring out, with Billie's help, how to do this so insurance will cover the costs. A compelling case has to be made.

Love, Dad.

December 17.

Dear Family and Friends,

Today we met with several folks involved with Adam's rehab—occupational, and physical therapists, the case manager, and by phone the social worker and Billie, the insurance representative. Goals were assessed and new goals set. Mostly, it was a time of celebrating Adam's accomplishments—he has, everyone agrees, come a long way. Rehab Without Walls will continue, but the hours per week will be cut to somewhere between 10 and 14. Adam seemed pleased with the meeting and especially with the praise he received—and his pleasure points toward an interesting conflict of interests. He wants to be finished with rehab, an interest shared by the insurance company, while Dawn Ann and I want him to receive all the help that he can possibly get. For us, prolonging rehab makes good sense.

December 20. Day 130.

Dear Adam:

Today is your mother's 55th birthday. Yesterday, after stopping at Checker Auto to get a snow and ice scraper, you and I went to the University Bookstore where we bought cards and then to lunch. At lunch you talked about your recovery, noting that none of the therapists you are working with quite know what to make out of you, that you don't fit any of the "normal" patterns for a brain injured person. When asked, you mentioned comments made by Meran, your speech therapist, who apparently reviewed symptoms with you, most notably crying, and reporting you didn't have "any of them." You talk about being normal "by May." I hope you are right although events of yesterday give me pause. Despite my best efforts, I could not get you to work out with hand weights yesterday, something you said you needed to do every other day. Nor did you ride the recumbent bike. I worry about what will happen when the therapists are gone, something you very much look forward to.

Lost Self

Dear Adam:

Last night I read the following words from Simon Crowe's book, *The Behavioural and Emotional Complications of Traumatic Brain Injury*: "It is hard to imagine what it must be like for an individual following the personal crisis and catastrophe that ensues as a result of a serious traumatic brain injury. The individual is confronted with a huge range of alterations in his or her normal functioning operating at the biological, psychological, and social levels.... All of these changes are also occurring to an individual who has just had a near death experience...and the not too surprising focus [follows:] 'Who am I?' and 'Why am I here?'" (p. 1). You often comment that no one could possible understand what you are going through if they haven't gone through it themselves. You are right, Adam. I cannot imagine what it must be like to wake up one day and not be who you recall yourself as being just the day before—discovering that weeks have actually passed, time without memory. Losing a self and losing all the abilities developed that define that self, or at least many of them, is impossible to imagine. Today I realized that as you sit and listen to the CD of you playing your music that what you must be doing is mourning the loss of yourself. This truly I cannot imagine.

I find myself wondering, What does it mean to recover fully? What is it you will have recovered? It seems that recovery might be confused with compensation. I cannot help but think about an article I read—re-read it last night—Charles Carver, Resilience and thriving: Issues, models and linkages, *Journal of Social Issues*, 54(2)—recently that discusses responses to adversity and to trauma. One of the subsections is entitled, "Trauma, thriving, and reorganization of the self." This is what you are facing, an unwanted and forced personal transformation and reorganization. No wonder you fixate on those few things that seem more than less stable—Clapton, Kirby, the ritual of drinking maté, that Argentinian tea that tastes like boiled grass to me. Surely this adds to your deep disappointment with some so-called friends who have proven themselves as only good in fair-weather. The goal isn't to merely be resilient—which, as Carver argues, is a homeostasis concept, a matter of getting back to something called "normal" (a word you often use), but to be better, to thrive, to be an Adam that is more than you were before but still you. This is my prayer.

We have now been told that Rehab Without Walls will only continue until you reach a set of functional goals—it's not about continuing improvement at all. I should have known this, but I didn't.

December 25, Christmas Day.

Dear Adam:

Having you alive, home, and healing made this a Christmas to remember.

We love you. Dad.

December 27.

Dear Adam:

Yesterday I took you shopping for speakers for the Zune you are giving to Kirby tomorrow for a late Christmas (she arrives in the morning). Foolishly, thinking that Circuit City would have a greater selection, I took you there first rather than doing what you wanted to do which was go to another store. You found some speakers at Circuit City but they were more than you wanted to spend and were, you insisted, more than a similar set would have been at another store. You are worrying about money, "Damn, I am poor," you said, and concerned about when you might be able to start working. You complained a great deal on our way home about your situation. I tried and tried to be encouraging, commenting multiple times on the miracle of your life, how grateful I am—we are—for your life and how you are making such good progress. On your part, you complained, said you wanted to be well "now," and insisted that no one could possibly understand what life is like for you. Well, we do understand more than you allow, but given your world of absolutes, a partial but good understanding simply doesn't count. Foolishly, I've tried to explain that other's lives have changed dramatically as well, that you are not the only one who has been put in a rough spot. Saying something like this is really stupid. I know better but I still comment. For example, I mentioned how having to quit school for the semester has actually put Rachel behind a full year. Your response: She was going to drop out anyway. Not true, but in your world that doesn't matter.

On Christmas Day as some of us sat in the sitting room chatting, we got onto the subject of TBI, how you use these letters in a funny way, but not wholly funny, to excuse your behavior when socially inappropriate. Not nice, but it was wonderful to be able to laugh and be silly.

> *Medical memo: "Many investigators agree that the most commonly reported personality change following TBI is increased irritability accompanied by the associated features of frustration, aggression, egocentricity, impulsiveness, impairment of judgment and insight, and inappropriate expression of affection. These changes seem to generate greater distress for patients in the period more than six months following the injury rather than in the acute stage."* [13]

December 31. New Years Eve.

Dear Adam:

It's a bit after 11 a.m. Heather from Rehab Without Walls just arrived.

I've been reading a book on the brain, *Your brain and your self: What you need to know* (written by Jacques Neirynck and translated by Laurence Garey). Using the book, last night I tried to figure out more precisely what part of your brain was injured. What I'm learning is that my effort is futile, that brain injuries are frequently diffuse not neatly localized—wiring problems manifest themselves in all sorts of strange ways. Your mother wondered if the swelling in your brain did damage and it may have. No way of knowing. You still have two sizeable scabs on your head, the result of the three bone flap surgeries and maybe of "swabbing." Last night before prayer you rubbed your head and checked the scabs, which you do periodically. Not having much hair—although you have a little soft fuzz across most of the area—really bothers you. You often mention that you are going to grow your hair long, and I don't blame you.

Even though having Kirby here has given you a lift, you continue to battle discouragement. I cannot really imagine how difficult this must be.

At dinner last night there was a bit of tension. I made the mistake of urging you to watch what you say, to make an effort to be less socially inappropriate. You immediately got defensive, and asked what you had done that was inappropriate. You had just let out an obnoxious burp, so I said, "What you just did, burping".

It's now 12:15, Heather has left and Maren has arrived. While waiting for Maren you said to your mother and me that it would have been easier if you had died. Your mother tried to get you to look at her, but you wouldn't, so she could tell you that we are glad you lived and love you. Right now words like these don't seem to matter much to you. You don't like your life, desperately wanting to be normal. As you see it, your life isn't worth living. But it will be, it will be.

> *Medical memo: "[The brain's] activity is not comparable to that of the central processor of a computer treating information sequentially according to a rigid program. The brain reacts as a whole, even if certain regions are specialized. The specific capacity of man to integrate a mass of information into a coherent vision of his environment, the place he occupies within it and the activity that he can pursue there, all stem from cooperation between these regions."*

"Area specialization in the brain is a concept that needs careful handling. When we compartmentalize the brain we focus our attention on detail, and may not be able to see the wood for the trees. Different areas have different functions, but they work together, just as a successful sports team relies less on the performance of a single player than on their capacity to collaborate." [14]

"I can do it, Dad"

January 4, 5:17, p.m.

Dear Adam:

Having Kirby here the past week has been a very good thing. Last night your mother and I went downstairs to see if you were ready for prayer. Both you and Kirby were exercising, each of you with your backs to one of the walls next to your bedroom door, knees bent, and she was counting to ten. She was encouraging, funny, and obviously determined. We've been worried a lot about what will happen when your therapists are finished: What will we do to get you to exercise?

As I've already mentioned, I've been reading Crowe's *The behavioural and emotional complications of traumatic brain injury*. Interesting and helpful. During church—shame on me—I read a section, chapter six, on "impaired self-awareness" which helped me better understand how difficult it is for you to see that your injury didn't only compromise your body but also your brain. Crowe notes that often there is an impairment of the ability to accurately perceive emotions as facially expressed (p. 135). Empathy also presents a problem. I need to remind myself that it's TBI that's to blame and be more patient.

Yesterday you, Mom and Kirby attended the traveling exhibit, "Body World," at the Leonardo science center. Apparently Kirby suggested you do this a couple of days before but you said you didn't want to go, that it would be too disturbing. She let it go, apparently knowing that the idea would return. So, on Friday night you mentioned that "you" should go, that Kirby would enjoy it. Your mom went on line and purchased tickets. I have to admit, I chose to not go, finding the very idea of these exposed bodies upsetting, wondering who these people were, what their lives were like, and what they would say if they could walk through the exhibit. You really enjoyed the time at the exhibit; your mother mentioned that you read and moved ahead from display to display rather quickly and on your own. After I picked you up you mentioned that standing in a crowd, and I guess it was very crowded, you nearly fell. I think you mentioned this because it proved so frightening.

The other day you mentioned that you are struggling with your faith. You wonder if your survival is simply a matter of luck. It isn't, Adam.

January 8, Thursday. Day 148.

Dear Adam:

You are walking without your cane and are moving much more quickly and with much greater self-assurance than even a few days ago. When we try to do things for you, you often protest, "I can do it, Dad." This is where all the talk about being an adolescent goes awry. The problem is that dependency is mistaken for immaturity and you are not immature, just revisiting some developmental issues like figuring out who you are under radically changed circumstances. You are a young man who possesses the experience and memories of a young man.

The other day I once again told you how I admire your courage. You strongly disagreed, saying that courage has nothing to do with it—I disagree, and strongly. "I do what I'm told," you say. In a sense you are compliant because you are resigned, signs of which are evident when you respond to a question about something, for instance, what you'd like to eat, by saying "whatever." But, the way I see it, you have a choice, you could sleep all the time, fight with us to be left alone, and wilt before the challenges you face. And you don't. I am proud of you, Adam, very proud.

Last night the Utah Jazz played New Orleans. Before the game you watched a movie with a friend. I came downstairs and asked you what sort of treat you wanted for the game. You pondered the question, gave up, said "surprise me," and just seconds after saying these words your face brightened, "E.L. Fudge cookies," you said. It took me a while to find them at the grocery store, but I did. Keebler Elves. It was fun to watch the game with you, patch in place over your left lens, and a few Wahoos! When I'm around you I drive you crazy, I know. I want to have you close, to touch you, a feeling that is very comforting. At one point during the game you moved away from me on the sofa. At another, you complained about how hot my hand was, noting, after I removed it from where it rested on you right side, "I can still feel it (the heat)...Nope, it's gone."

Yesterday you had two therapy sessions. With Heather you rode the bus to Wasatch Elementary School and worked some more in your mother's library. Later, with Lisa, among other things, you rode the recumbent bike for 15 minutes at a 20 setting—something I don't think I could do, which seems to please you. You've stuck to your guns and are adding a minute a day. We hope this continues.

January 12.

Dear Adam:

Today, Monday, marks five months to the day of your accident. It is also Grandpa Bullough's 83rd birthday. Tonight we'll go to my folks' home for cake and ice cream.

Friday you had two appointments, the first at 10 a.m. to have your teeth cleaned, something that hasn't been done for quite some time. On the way to the dentist's office you complained, saying that if problems turned up you weren't going to do anything about them. You said that you had had enough of being worked on. Happily, after your checkup, the dentist said, "Everything looks good." I was amazed. Five months of not flossing, and everything looks good!

Later your mother and I took you for an appointment with Dr. Parkin, our family physician, to see what needed to be done with the blood clot filter that was placed in your body sometime in early September, I believe. We tried to reassure you that having the filter removed isn't a big deal, but you weren't having any of it. I can't blame you: Who wants to have surgery even as an "outpatient" after what you have gone through? Tomorrow I take you to LDS Hospital where a radiologist will take the pictures necessary to know what to do. At first you were pleased to know that some people simply never have the filters removed. You seemed to change your mind, however, after I commented that leaving a foreign object in your body is unwise and after Dr. Parkin commented that sometimes they cause problems, clot up and impede blood flow. Not good.

Dr. Parkin looked at your head and said everything looks great, then said, smiling, you don't want to go "bald." Good point. The scabs are gone and your hair is growing back in most places. Last night Seth felt your head and asked if you felt anything. You said that you didn't. Time will tell how much feeling returns.

Your mother keeps Caringbridge going and reads others' journal entries. She came into the Study and said that another hospital friend has died. We are not telling you this. Paul was in room 16 of the SICU, your room, the "Lucky room," we were told. His brain started hemorrhaging again and nothing could be done. I feel so badly for his wife and young son. Thank goodness they had a child.

January 14. Day 155.

Today we had the last of the consultations with the Rehab Without Walls folks. You passed all the goals that were set by and for you. Today is exactly two months since you came home. As I said, I misunderstood how RWW works, believing that, as Billie, from our insurance company, said, as "long as you make progress" the insurance would cover your rehab. It turns out what she really meant was that the moment you reach a set of goals, they are done. Now, the question is, what do we do with the 25 outpatient visits they'll pay for? (with a $25 co-pay, which surprised you). Lisa, who really has been wonderful, is working on setting things up with a person who can help with your balance. We shall miss her.

Yesterday the filter was removed from your vena cava artery. Good to have it out. The actual procedure took about 15 minutes but we spent nearly four hours at the hospital.

Your mother made airline reservations for you and Rachel to return to California in mid-February.

Friendship and Family

January 17.

Kirby and Emmely arrived from California. A long drive.

January 19.

Dear Adam:

Tomorrow is Barack Obama's inauguration as 44th president. Amazing.

Early this morning your mother came into the bedroom. "The girls are leaving," she said. I hurriedly got up, put on some clothing and dashed out front to find her scraping the ice from Kirby's car windows. I got my scraper and helped. We didn't realize they planned to leave for home so early. We're grateful Kirby and Emmely came for the weekend. Their visit gave you a real lift. They arrived about 1 a.m. Saturday morning. You and Kirby talked until about 3 a.m. this morning so I'm doubly glad that Emmely came with Kirby who must have been exhausted when they left. Your mother felt badly because she planned on cooking waffles for breakfast, thinking they weren't going to leave until a bit later in the morning. Their decision was wise, however, based on anticipation of a huge motorcade moving from Las Vegas to Los Angeles.

You came into the bedroom where I was reading this morning and reported that Dr. Chang sent you an email. You'd written to him and he responded, signing "Bill Chang." You mentioned that you might want to get a t-shirt for him to wear and discussed possible things to put on it. We discussed the possibility of writing: "I saved Adam Bullough." You commented that you'd need three of these, one for Kirby, one for Dr. Chang and one for Dr. Massoudi. Then, you said that you weren't certain you had enough money for so many shirts. Money matters worry you.

About 4:30 this evening I went downstairs to see if you wanted something to eat. I knew you hadn't eaten lunch. I crossed the room and looked into the dark to see you sitting, immobile, on the couch facing the tv. "Adam, Adam." No answer. No movement. Feeling the first signs of terror come over me, I walked closer and touched you, saying, "Adam." You opened your eyes! What a relief! It may seem silly, but I check on you periodically, still worrying, as parents do, about whether or not you are all right. I know you get sick of me touching you, but each touch gives just a hint of reassurance that you are well...and with us.

January 21.

Dear Adam:

Today Corina Ayla took you to Costco. We are so very grateful for all she does for and with you. I tried and tried to get you to go swimming Monday and Tuesday and also have tried and tried to get you to ride the recumbent bike today but without success. Your mother and I remain very worried. Last night, late, I went downstairs to say "goodnight" and heard you playing the guitar for a moment and then a spate of swearwords. Kirby was on the phone listening, which saddened me. You said that playing only frustrates you—but if you don't play, then you won't be able to play, and that's the choice before you. Your frustration and depression are certainly understandable but I hope and pray they do not defeat you.

January 22. Day 163.

Dear Adam:

Today we met with Dr. Ryser who urged us to get things set up for you with work, which we need to do. We shared our lingering concerns about your eyes—double vision—and your left side weakness, particularly with your hand. He spoke briefly about the challenges of getting "higher level skills," like playing the guitar, back and also mentioned that if your vision hasn't shown significant signs of improvement in a month we need to set up an appointment with an optometrist, saying that there are [thick prism] glasses that might help. I think you found these words discouraging. Earlier today, and trying to be encouraging, I read to you from a book, *The Compassionate Brain* by Gerald Huther: Pointing toward a study of the brains of London taxi drivers that showed the neuronal networks connected to the work of finding one's way around a place like London became progressively bigger the longer they drove— "The brain researchers....were quite amazed to discover how great the use-dependent malleability of the human brain is. If we take their findings to the logical conclusion, the implication is that the brain takes on the form of how it is used" (p. 85). Of course, Huther is not writing about injured brains but healthy ones. Still, I find the message hopeful.

The battle with discouragement continues, even as you asserted to Dr. Ryser that you are not depressed. Your frustration comes out sometimes as anger. The possibility of you not being able to play the guitar or run freely troubles me deeply and I know it adds to your ongoing struggle with faith and with God.

January 23.

Dear Family and Friends, (Dawn Ann writing)

Grandpa Mortensen picked up Adam this afternoon. They are having a sleep over. Adam's idea. They watched Charlie Chaplin's movie, "The Gold Rush," and are now just hanging out. Dawn Ann got teary as she realized this was the first day since August 13th that she has not been with Adam. Bob and Dawn Ann are having Adam withdrawals!

January 24.

Dear Adam:

Tonight the two of us watched the Jazz lose to Cleveland on televison. At half time you took off your eye patch and glasses and expressed your frustration about not being able to see, suggesting that we schedule an appointment with an optometrist sooner than the month Dr. Ryser suggested. One of the challenges is that you have difficulty telling if your eyes are improving or not.

Tonight I read multiple times the glossary of terms in one of the "brain" books I read this week. The more I read the more amazed I become that we have avoided nearly all of the terrible things that might have happened given the nature and extent of your injury. I cannot help but think about how really bad things might have been.

"You're having a great recovery"

January 27. Day 168.

Dear Adam:

Shortly after 8 a.m. yesterday you had a blood test at the hospital and at 8:35 we met with Dr. Caine, a neuropsychologist, to begin a cognitive evaluation. Having to get up early and anticipating the day upset you; you were on edge. It promised, you said, to be a colossal "waste of your time." You claimed not to be nervous, but clearly you were. I know I was. The first hour you especially hated since it involved Dr. Caine asking questions of us, you, your mother and me. Usually you do not like to hear what we have to say. Your mother went back to work once testing began, and I dashed to Costco next door, then read and waited. Following lunch we returned for more testing. During lunch you seemed to be in a pretty good mood, even laughing about some test items. You, once again, had proven yourself to yourself. Anticipating the possibility of being told I have some serious cognitive deficits would really worry me—in fact, I didn't sleep all night in part because of concern about what we might hear about you even as I believed the report would prove positive. It did. Very positive. After the afternoon session of testing you and I met with Dr. Caine who said the following: "You are having a great recovery!" There are no major weaknesses, a little forgetting and some very mild fluency issues which likely will pass. Your double vision, he said, very well might contribute to these problems. Again, he said, your "recovery has been great!" On the way to lunch you described Dr. Caine as "all business," and for him to be so very positive given his affect and professional demeanor seemed especially significant. In the morning he told us—you, me, your mother—that he believed it important to provide honest feedback, even when the news isn't good.

After discussing the "quantitative" results of your assessment, based on the tests—which showed you to be "normal" (a state you long for), Dr. Caine turned to the "qualitative" and more praise followed. He said that you seem able to work your way around problems such that the effects of your injury are not "a big deal." You are even, he noted, compensating well for your vision problem. "Balance and dexterity can continue to improve," he said. "Try to be patient." He urged patience multiple times, stating that you are still relatively early into your recovery.

Dr. Caine mentioned that you have some weakness in your right as well as your left hand, something I've noticed particularly when you eat with a fork.

By way of summary, he said, "Do things that keep the brain active." "Turning on different areas of the brain helps healing." He urged you to "read, write, and speak"—"read, talk, write," suggesting that you read materials you like. Dr. Caine urged you to return to school slowly, taking a couple of classes and assessing how well things go.

Just before leaving Dr. Caine said that he had read the materials on your case in preparation for the session. Like so many others, he said that you surprised him. Given the severity of your injury, he had expected much more serious deficits. You left the meeting, as did I, very pleased. I appreciated his willingness to answer questions, and I had quite a few. I cannot help but compare our experience with him to that had with the neuropsychologist at Mission Hospital, the one who borrowed the book. He even answered my questions about how the cerebellum operates—he said it serves relay functions and that this may account for the weaknesses on your left—and also right—sides. The messages sent are interrupted.

After the sessions with Dr. Caine and although you were tired, you were in a very good mood. We spent the evening at Josh and Vorn's apartment playing Wii. You and I even played. Boxing. I had no idea what I was doing. No doubt you boxed double opponents! Shortly after arriving home from Josh's you went downstairs. Returning upstairs you happily announced, "I made it up the stairs without touching the walls."

Love, Dad.

January 28.

Dear Adam:

This morning, and it's very early, I've been lying in bed thinking about our experience with the neuropsychologist at Mission Hospital. As I've thought about what she said my feelings toward her have sharpened and become even more negative than they were before. Several of Dr. Caine's comments got me thinking. At the time of our meeting with her I was put off by her dismissive and arrogant manner, how she made judgments about you and about us without ever having spoken to you or to us. Yet she spoke confidently when she said that we needed to understand that you were like a "bright ten-year-old." Of course, she was wrong about this and on many fronts. Her advice was mostly foolish but said with all the weight her Ph.D. could carry. She mentioned you needed to recover yourself, but this singly important point got lost in other chatter, talk that we'd be raising you all over again. It's taken me some time but I've come to understand at least to some degree your struggle—that your sense of yourself was shattered, that you were groping, anxiously reaching for some familiar bits of the Adam you knew and you were not finding many. Suddenly the very independent, proud and handsome young man you were was gone, replaced by a feeble and very dependent stranger needing help with even the most simple of tasks, peeing, sitting up, eating. No wonder you got agitated, found nothing funny, were easily frightened, and often unforgivingly demanding. Why didn't she say this? Instead, her central message was that you were a child. You were not and are not. You were a disoriented and injured young man needing help to recapture as much of your competent self as possible and needing a hansel of hope. At the time, I didn't know that I should not have believed her about this, even though I knew then she didn't have a clue about you. I should have known she knew even less about your future. Now I could push back, and insist on being heard. But then, in my desperate need for any kind of reassurance that you'd be all right, I played into her professional need to speak with authority. I didn't know she didn't know and I was afraid to ask.

It is now about 4:30 p.m. The visit with Dr. Jensen, your neurosurgeon, went very well. You seemed pleased. He is a remarkable man. I appreciated how willing he was to respond to some of the questions that have perplexed me these many weeks. On August 21st we were told about the four "dead spots" or "strokes" in your brain. These were terms that were used to describe your injury, and hearing them used for the first time ever so long ago made my heart sink. He said that he doesn't pay a lot of attention to talk of this kind, that it usually comes from radiologists and they don't have a particularly good understanding of the brain. "Dead" doesn't necessarily mean "dead," he said, and that "stroke" means many different things as well. He said these spots were described in many ways, including "defuse axonal injury" (a term I actually understand). I asked him about why the section of bone was removed from your temporal lobe and not elsewhere. He said that surgeons like to make as big an opening as possible to relieve swelling, and this is a good place. Additionally, he said that had you been bleeding there, which you apparently weren't, that would also be a determining factor. I asked if the place of an injury and the need to manipulate the head during surgery had a part in the decision. He said it could. Finally, I asked questions about the cerebellum. I really appreciated what he said, and especially how willing he was to teach us.

The meeting started with Dr. Jensen saying to you, "Oh, you look great." He was delighted with what had happened and joked about how well patients do when he does little. He was so confident that everything was as it should be that he almost forgot to look at the brain scan. When he did, his initial judgment was confirmed. With the scan on the screen he answered a few additional questions, and each answer underscored how well you are healing. He made a point of saying that in his work with brain tumor patients he has sometimes had to remove large portions of the cerebellum, a primitive part of the brain (I said, "the reptilian part," which seemed to surprise him—"Yes," he said). Such patients can have full recoveries, he said. He was confident given the nature and extent of your injury that you'll heal completely. I made a comment about the nature and challenges of his work. After mentioning that he "lost" his father (age 78) three weeks ago and the limits of his own understanding of his father's health problems (the father worked at Geneva Steel and had lung problems that made it impossible for him to fight off a case of pneumonia) he spoke a bit about his experience as a surgeon, of having a couple of times made a call that saved a person but left them in a vegetative state. Experiences of this kind troubled him, deeply. He mentioned his father because this experience put him on the other side, the family side, of illness. He knew and appreciated the difficulties families face when trying to make good decisions for their ill loved ones and how difficult it is to get helpful guidance and useful information. He said that he wondered what he had done to the families of the people who had a poor recovery. But, the highs of his work are wonderful, he said. Obviously, your recovery offers one of those life-affirming highs. He seemed pleased when we told him you would be visiting Mission Hospital soon. This is important, he said.

January 30.

Dear Family and Friends, (Dawn Ann writing)

Adam came to [the school this morning]. Dawn Ann received a teaching award that was presented before the entire student body. The highlight for her was looking at her family and seeing Adam sitting there, healing and growing stronger... The other highlight was the excitment of the children seeing Adam. They do love him.

Dear Adam:

You spent most of the day with my parents. Dad picked you up from the balance clinic and brought you home. He was really pleased at how you were able to tie flies even though, he said, the two of you did more talking than tying. This, of course, is probably just what you need. As Dr. Caine said—writing, reading and *talking*. It's increasingly obvious that you need to spend more time away from home and busy.

January 31. Day 172.

Dear Adam:

I just did a Google search on cerebromalacia. After our meeting with Dr. Jensen I emailed him asking for the word that he used to describe the "spots" on your brain: encephalomalacia led to cerebromalacia. I found an entry that was helpful, a response by an MD to a question: "Cerebromalacia (I often use the term encephalomalacia) refers to loss of brain tissue... Basically, the injured brain tissue was reabsorbed and the resulting MRI or CT scan has a particular appearance identified as encephalomalacia. It is a descriptive term rather than the name of a disease per se... [T]his just reflects a change of appearance of dead brain tissue rather than any new pathologic process... From your description, I expect the encephalomalacia to appear in the occipital lobes (the person being written about went blind)... I hope this helps..." So, I guess these are the spots but, as Dr. Jensen said, using these words and descriptions doesn't really reveal much.

A final item: Today you went to the Farmington Bay Water Fowl Management Preserve with Mom. You saw two bald eagles perching in a dead tree. As your mom said, "Pretty cool." On the way you discovered something rather surprising. If you tilt your head downward but look outward your double vision disappears. We wonder what this means. After all the time you spent in the hospital and having had so many disappointments, you cannot imagine that this is a good sign. You'll wait and see and it is one or another expert that will make the judgment. Expert opinion remains the only opinion you are interested in other than your own.

On Healing

Dear Adam:

We frequently have brief talks which often end in frustration. Your mother and I do not know how to help you deal with your feelings of frustration and persistent anger. You are discouraged and there are hints of you becoming increasingly resigned to the possibility that you will never play the guitar or play soccer again at anything approaching a level that is enjoyable. Last night you commented that you have tried and tried to play the Cream song, "Sunshine of your love," but can't. Somehow I think you got it in your mind, and you aren't alone in this, that the healing of a brain is like the healing of a bodily wound. Of course, it's not. A crossed left eye and double vision are constant reminders that, as you say, you are not "healing fast enough." You've commented to your mom that you want to know why God doesn't heal you even as your faith diminishes.

Last night you said, "I've had everything taken from me." Not everything, Adam, not everything. You are alive, smart, and healing.

February 6.

Dear Adam:

We spent this morning with Dr. Ballard (a physical therapist) at the University's balance clinic who did an evaluation of your balance. Interesting. He began by saying that your healing is dependent on you, that no one can do it for you. He checked you out by tapping you all over to check your reflexes: knees, feet, arms. He tested your strength. Here are a few of the comments made: The balance system is composed of three things—"vision, inner ear and body knowledge: we interact with the world through our feet." Balance is "a matter of keeping the belly button centered over the feet." This helps explain why you walk with your feet wide apart. As your vision improves, he believes your balance will improve, but vision only contributes a small part to your difficulties with balance. To better understand what is going on he conducted several tests including a "Sensory Organization Test". This test provided data that helps pinpoint the sources of balance difficulty: vision, inner ear or body knowledge. You were placed in a harness and "hung" in a tall three-sided box of sorts, the open end is where Dr. Ballard stood close behind you, just in case something happened. He carefully positioned your feet and then directed your actions. You stood on a plate that tilted as did the box itself at certain points in the testing. There were six different "conditions," including open and closed eyes. You were told to "stand quietly" and then the conditions were changed; after 20 seconds a computer scored the results eventually producing an overall "equilibrium score." In all, you "fell" five times (out of six on the inner ear tests). From there we went back into the exam room where you were hooked up to a kind of face mask that blacked out your vision. The mask was connected to a screen that allowed Dr. Ballard to see how your eyes (he only tested your right eye) responded to different conditions, including following the rapid movement of your head from side to side and up and down twenty times. At one point someone came into the room and borrowed a board, about two feet by two feet, that had a black and white checkerboard pattern on it. I don't know what it is used for. Dr. Ballard remarked, often head injury people are "visually sensitive." To this you said something that was new to me, that "patterns" give you difficulty.

All along the way Dr. Ballard explained everything he was doing and often why he was doing it, from getting into the three-sided box to walking a 25 foot line down the adjacent hallway. At the conclusion of the testing he said that to his surprise, yours is primarily an "inner ear" problem but this may not be a problem with the inner ear per se but with your brain's ability to utilize information from your inner ear to maintain balance. He said that you did very well with your feet and were a bit low, but not really bad, with your eyes—which he thought remarkable given your double vision.

You were given a written set of exercises that you are supposed to do every day. When I reminded you of this after you rested at home you got very angry with me, saying that you didn't nag me about my Pepsi drinking so why should I nag you about doing these exercises? You are to walk 30 minutes a day, march in place, stand in a corner and do a series of eye-open and eye-closed exercises, among other activities.

Today, while reading and doing my minutes on the recumbent bike, I ran across this statement: "Of all the discrete emotions, anger is the affect that has been most consistently associated with health impairment." (From a chapter written by N. Consedine and C. Magai in the *Handbook of Adult Development and Learning*, edited by C. Hoare, p. 139). I need to remind myself that there are reasons for you being angry. As you put it, you've had many of the activities you most love doing "taken away from you." God gets the blame. I suppose God is a better object of your anger than blaming yourself for not wearing a helmet. I need to be more understanding of what you are feeling even as I need to continue to insist you do the work necessary to heal. We cannot let you off the hook.

You spent some time late this afternoon with Seth. You went with him to buy a new motorcycle helmet. I appreciate how Seth is making time for you. You spent much of yesterday with my parents, tying flies with Dad and playing games with both Dad and Mom. On my way home from Provo, on the 6th South freeway exit into the city, I noticed it was getting dark and realized that I'd better phone to see if you were home. Dad doesn't like to drive when it is dark. You were still with my parents, so I made my way to their place to get you. On the way your mother phoned. She had a flat tire. Thank goodness Joshua was able to help her. At my folks I sat and watched the three of you have a wonderful time playing a card game, then we met Mom for dinner and drove home. A long day.

Money Matters and Much Kindness

February 11.

Dear Adam:

Today is Wednesday. Tomorrow I turn 60.

I spent Monday morning in the insurance company's downtown offices meeting with Yvette, the accountant assigned to our case. It was a difficult morning. On Saturday I received a letter from the Trauma Group threatening us, saying that our account is significantly overdue and within 10 days would be sent to a collection agency. Some weeks before we were supposed to be sent an updated bill but none came. After Yvette spoke with the accounts person for the Group and explained that the bills are being worked on we were given an extension to the end of the month. Apparently, and I don't understand this at all, DMBA, our insurance company, has hired another company to work on our account to find alternative contractors than First Health of California. The hope is that this company will figure out ways for reducing payments. The Trauma Group is not contracted so we are left with quite a bit to pay beyond the amount DMBA pays. It angers me that we were not given a choice of who we would work with in the hospital, that, in effect, we were assigned the most expensive physicians. This said, such matters are trivial in the immediate aftermath of an injury like yours. Still, I can't understand how one physician could charge us for 19 $300 visits nor can I understand how it is that many of these visits involve differing payment amounts from the insurance company. Nothing makes sense.

The bill for October 27th, the day of your flap surgery, was $199,400.74. Staggering.

Over the weekend Robert Ramirez, the volunteer who was so very kind to us at Mission Hospital, phoned to see how we were doing. Your mother spoke with him. He mentioned that Tuesday (yesterday) there was to be a meeting during which patient issues would be addressed. After the meeting with Yvette I'd planned to send an email to him about our concerns but forgot. Stupid.

Yesterday, after taking your mother to work early (we had a dandy of a snow storm and since her new tires haven't arrived she's driving on a donut following the flat) and fiddling around for a while I cooked you a Popeye eggie, and began the effort to get you to do your balance exercises. When you do them you count the requisite 20 seconds but your counting is rather fast. (In contrast, I cheat in the other direction as I look at my wristwatch.) The result of your speedy counting is that you finish quickly and, no doubt, get less benefit.

Yesterday I did some of the balance exercises with you. I couldn't stand long on one leg, either leg, which surprised you. Mom has exercised with you. We're hoping that while you are in California (you leave Friday evening) that Kirby will do them with you. Somehow we have got to get you working more consistently and harder.

Around noon yesterday after taking Rachel to school I took you to your mother's school. You were very angry about going, saying that "you don't have a choice." How you hate having so little control over your life! You stayed a while at the school and helped your mother in the library but soon left, walking home. Your mom pointed out that she didn't care that you were angry, only that you walked home (one of your exercises is to walk 30 minutes a day and at an increasingly rapid pace). I guess it took about 40 minutes for you to get home.

February 18. Day 190.

Dear Adam:

It's Wednesday morning, early, and I'm at work in Provo. Yesterday evening you, Kirby, Rachel and Matt had dinner with Dr. Chang in California.. I spoke to you afterwards. You said it was a wonderful evening, that you now are on a "hugging basis" with Dr. Chang. Remember, Adam, I hugged him first! After dinner he rushed back to the hospital to "do a procedure" leaving you and Kirby (Rachel and Matt had to leave earlier). You mentioned that he really likes your music, said you should get a "producer," and that his favorite song is "Going to California." After we spoke I was so pleased all I could do was smile.

Hopefully, Kirby is working you hard while you are away.

Yesterday I met with Yvette, the accountant, again. She's been wonderful, even as I continue to be just a bit overwhelmed. After our meeting I returned home, did more organizing of bills, paid a few, and in the process realized that there are still several Trauma Group bills outstanding. I found these just as I was beginning to think that we'd finished with them. In any case, the outfit DMBA hired to find alternative ways of reducing the billing— or put differently, of finding insurers to contract with that the Group accepts—apparently has paid off. There were several additional bills that are now taken care of. On my part, I simply don't know where we stand since I am not party to the ongoing interaction between the insurers and the providers. A side note: I found out that we have been charged around $4,300 for a private room in Acute Rehab even though we never requested one and DMBA doesn't cover the costs. I phoned the hospital and was shuffled around to four people, maybe five, before I was told, "I'll have the nurse check on this."

February 20.

Dear Adam:

Your mother and I just got home from a Mardi Gras gathering attended by several of the folks associated with her school. As we were driving home, Sue Mordin phoned and reported she and Diana had a wonderful time at breakfast with you, Rachel and Matt. From the restaurant you had a view of the ocean and could see dolphins swimming in the distance. I spoke with you a couple of times today. The first time was shortly after you and Kirby visited Dr. Massoudi at his office. It was a short visit, you said, but you seemed very happy. Once again, you were told you are a miracle. I asked how having this said about you made you feel, "Good." I know, a stupid question to ask. Dr. Massoudi checked your head and, you said, he seemed quite pleased. Later we talked just as you were leaving Mission Hospital after visiting many of those who cared for you. I wish I could have been there. I imagine seeing you was uplifting—I still marvel when I think about how demanding the work is that these people do. Daniel and Christine weren't there, but many of the nurses were as was Dr. Sarafian, who you also saw on Monday. All in all, you had a very good day. It's wonderful to feel your enthusiasm.

I miss you.

"I don't care"

Dear Adam:

Last night you, Seth, and Grandma and Grandpa Bullough attended the Jazz game. These were the tickets we purchased for Mom for Christmas. I made stew and they came over for dinner before the game. I then drove the four of you to the arena. The game was a slaughter, with the Hawks not giving the Jazz much of a challenge.

Before leaving for the game I mentioned to you that you might want to take your cane. "NO!", you protested. But, when the time came to leave you took it. You were worried about the crowds and being jostled and falling, even suggesting that you wanted to go to the game late to avoid them. Dad said you used the cane, especially on the escalators. I'm glad.

At home, after the game, we chatted. You said that you didn't use your eye patch while watching the game. The distance between where you were sitting and the court was so great that the two images of the game caused by your double vision where quite far apart, and you knew which one was "real." One image, you said, was mostly off in the crowd. The strain of keeping the images separated got to you at times, you said, and you found it necessary to periodically shake your head to get your eyes back to where you could see. You looked exhausted.

You remain very angry toward God, wondering why He hasn't healed you. Nothing I or we say changes your view. Seeing you battle with depression breaks my heart. One of your last comments last night, said just as I was leaving to go upstairs, was this: "If you had to deal with this, you'd have already committed suicide." These words were very upsetting. I got into my exercise clothes and went upstairs, even though it was late, and rode the recumbent bike and watched "Last of the Summer Wine" on PBS.

This morning I went downstairs and asked you if you'd like to walk Layla. You were dark, grumpy, sitting on the table in front of the TV where you seemed to be programming something, a video game I think. You remarked that you were going to Corina's to talk in Spanish and drink maté (thank goodness for her). You said that all I do is talk about therapy. You make a good point. As I was about to leave I noticed that on the right side of your head you had some skin stuck in your hair. When I asked if you wanted it removed, you remarked, "I don't care." When you wash your hair you just brush the right side and back of your head. Last night at dinner you said your head "hurt," suggesting as your mother said that the nerves are healing in the skin. She's probably right.

I wish I knew how to be helpful, Adam.

February 26, Thursday.

Dear Adam:

Today the two of us walked to Wasatch Elementary School to see your mother at work—and to walk. It's about a mile and one half, and you were worn out. Rather than wait for an hour or more for your mother to be able to take us home, you phoned Rachel who met us part way. Once home you immediately fell asleep on the downstairs couch.

> *Memory (age 14, May): "You set the school record for the mile run and were invited to represent [the school] at the district track meet."*

March 2. Day 202.

Dear Adam:

I spent this morning lining up therapy appointments for you. You have an appointment on March 16th with Dr. Smith who specializes in voice rehab and on April 6th with Dr. Katz a neuro-ophthalmologist. When I gave you the news you were still lying in bed. You got angry, complained that the eye appointment should have been set up earlier and said, when I mentioned that we needed a referral from Dr. Ryser to get these appointments, "I don't believe it." It's true that I cannot possibly understand how frustrating your double vision is but I wish you could understand how hard we are working to help you. It took nearly an hour and half this morning and several calls to get these appointments set up and the related insurance issues clarified. I worry. You seem to think that getting to an eye specialist will produce a quick solution to your double vision when, like everything else connected to your healing, nothing, absolutely nothing, comes fast nor easily.

March 3.

Dear Adam:

Quite a day. The mail came and, as usual, there were several "This Is Not a Bill" statements from the insurance company, just a reporting of what has been paid on a specific bill or cluster of bills. As usual I went through them, lined things up by number, and concluded, happily, that the third party hired to find a way around the Trauma Group's refusal to accept our insurance as full payment was successful. Then, while working in the Study, the phone rang. Galiana from the Group saying that we would be getting a large bill, that DMBA had fouled everything up, and that despite multiple phone calls and letters nothing had improved, the Trauma Group was not contracted and we had to pay. I phoned Yvette at DMBA, who returned my call. Yvette knew nothing about what was said, hadn't received any information, but would listen to the phone message I mentioned Galiana said she left and get back to me. She did. She has to speak with her supervisor. So, more waiting.

Seems like "It's raining"

March 4.

Dear Adam:

Today we had another session with Dr. Ballard, Jim, as he insists on being called. He's great! Using data he gathered from your first visit, he made comparisons between your performance then and today on a variety of activities—from rising and walking quickly around a small red plastic cone and returning to a sitting position to walking heel to toe and standing on one leg. He timed everything. Walking around the cone: 8.9 improving to 7.1 seconds. Standing on your left leg, eyes closed: 2-3 seconds then, 8 seconds now. (In fact, you really couldn't do this the first time.) As you began to lose your balance you did what Dr. Ballard described, complimenting you, as a "Chuck Berry Move," working your foot side to side to stay upright. You had a little difficulty walking toe to heel. He said you are making "good progress," and mentioned that the key is to keep working but at increasingly challenging tasks: "We improve our balance by challenging it," he said. Today was your first day on "dyna disks" which are two oval, green, plastic, inflated things about a foot in diameter that a person stands on which require subtle shifts to maintain balance. After you finished, I stood on them—not easy. Dr. Ballard said that you are to begin walking heel to toe five times a day, and continue to walk on increasingly uneven surfaces. We need to get some foam to help with the task of standing on one leg, eyes open and closed. You are supposed to do a lot more eyes closed activities as well.

We made appointments for the next few weeks on Wednesdays. Amy Black will be your therapist. On the way to the session you mentioned that you'd found one of the drum sticks you made before your mission. This got me thinking, and I asked if drumming was something you would like to do. As we talked, I realized that this is a good idea, that drumming would work your body in all sorts of wonderful ways—and perhaps offer an outlet for your frustrated musical interests. Dr. Ballard mentioned that it's important to make therapy as fun as possible—you kicked around a soccer ball for a while today. Drumming certainly fits here. He even said that in the future you'd get outside for some activities. So, when we got in the car and you asked if I was serious about the possibility of getting a drum set, I said I was but that we would need to talk with your mother. We did. She agreed. And the order is in, an early birthday present. You've made a commitment to play and seem quite excited about it, commenting as you worked on the computer to find what was available, "I love drumming."

> *Memory (age 15, October): "You've been doing incredibly well in indoor soccer—a great sport! Today you came home happy despite the team losing 7 to 3. You said the other team was terrific and you were pleased with how well you and the team played. By the way, you've scored one or two goals in every game, twice with your left foot."*

> *Memory, (age 13, November): "A cold and wet day. Despite a hard fought loss, Sam Alba, your coach, was thrilled with your play, complimenting you: 'That's what soccer is all about!'"*

March 7. Day 206.

Dear Family and Friends, (Dawn Ann writing)

This evening Dawn Ann and Adam went to see Bobbi McFerrin in concert. Fabulous. Adam did great going up and down all the stairs and maneuvering through the crowds. We loved the music. McFerrin involved dancers, musicians, and drama students from the University [in his performance]. Dawn Ann sat in the concert [listening] and thought of how wonderful [it is] to have Adam sitting next to her.

March 8.

Dear Adam:

I had to speak in church today. Here's my penultimate paragraph:

"So, what good has come of Adam's injury? Adam continues to battle depression and dark feelings of abandonment of a very few people he thought his friends, and he struggles to regain himself and his body. I'm having difficulty reconnecting with work; many of my earlier activities seem less important, even stupid. Dawn Ann is a year behind in her library endorsement program. Rachel lost a year of school (but, in fairness, I should mention that she gained a California boyfriend). And, I spend time dealing with billing agencies and the accountant assigned to our case by the insurance company. But... having experienced God's grace, we have become a stronger family, more trusting, forgiving, more determined to care for and love one another. I think we are kinder and I believe we are better people. The price for these outcomes has been high, but the blessings bounteous. For one thing, we better understand the Father's feelings watching his beloved Son's suffering."

March 9, Monday.

Dear Adam:

This morning I went downstairs to see if you wanted a Popeye eggie. You wanted to sleep—it was about 10:30. So, I let you sleep, and later made you a pastrami "Reuben". You were in the bathroom, moving quickly because, you said, you needed to phone Kirby before she went to work. The past few days have been difficult for you because you and Kirby had a misunderstanding—she took something you said to mean that you didn't want to "be with her." You've done some scrambling to try to convince her that this isn't what you meant. When cooked, I brought the sandwich downstairs, but you were talking to Kirby and told me you'd "come upstairs." While you were eating the sandwich I asked you when you wanted to go walking, "maybe later." Well, later came around 2 p.m. when you came into the bedroom, dressed. I was reading. I bundled up and we went outside where a cold wind was blowing and it was snowing lightly. You were cold, buttoned up your sweater, and then decided you didn't want to walk, after all. I couldn't even get you to go to the end of our block. On the way back inside I foolishly mentioned that when you were in the hospital you did three hours of therapy a day. At these words you got upset and stormed into the house saying, "Now, I won't do any [exercises] at all!" "I'm not getting better!" In frustration, as you charged downstairs, I remarked, "Now, that is smart."

It is now 3:20 and you came into the Study, saying, "It's a good thing we didn't walk, have you looked out there, it's also raining." It's not. Just a little snow melt. But it is snowing harder.

March 12 (seven months to the day since you fell).

Dear Adam:

At your appointment today at the balance clinic you were retested on the "Balance Master." This is the machine that surrounds you while you are strapped in and creates various conditions to which you must adjust to maintain your balance, else you "fall." You did better this time, falling twice—last time you fell six times, really being unable to maintain your balance under the "eyes-closed" condition. Throughout you favored your right leg, your stronger leg.

"Stand quietly with eyes closed." Condition: "Eyes closed, sway referenced support." You fell. This involves the floor tilting front to back. Between the first and second series Amy coached you on using your toes, ankles, and hips. The coaching helped. She redid condition five, "Eyes closed, sway reference support." "I want you to really concentrate on your toes." You fell. "Stand quietly with your eyes closed." As the machine shifted, she said, "toes down, toes down...pay attention to your toes." Condition six: "Eyes open, sway referenced surround and support." Again, you fell. "Toes down, toes down." The surround moves upward and tilts toward you. The second time you had three falls. Amy then did a third "eyes closed" test, condition five and then six again. After reviewing the testing, and noting your improvement, she produced an exercise check-off sheet. I should mention that when reviewing your performance she said that brain injuries often make it difficult to judge exercise levels, and she urged you to push yourself. You said you likely wouldn't keep an exercise log, so this is the reason for her producing the sheet. She showed you the exercises she wants you to do which include stretching, strength and cardio-vascular activities. As you did the exercises you commented, "I'm so inflexible." She also talked about working the toes and your ankles to help your balance. On the way home you said you didn't feel well, that you were very "tired."

March 14, Saturday.

Dear Adam:

After some errands, I picked up a couple of sandwiches at Subway. Getting home I called to you to come and eat. I wasn't certain what you liked other than turkey and ham, so I purchased two different sandwiches—turkey and ham and Spicy Italian. Looking at what I bought, you got upset, refused to eat, and walked away, grumbling, "I don't like pickles." My fault, I forgot. I got pretty irritated. Removing the pickles, you then graciously ate half of the turkey and ham sandwich.

I just walked into the house. Shortly you will arrive. We were out walking. I had asked if you wanted to go for a walk. "I have no choice," you said, and grumpily got up and ready to go. As we walked around the side of the house I glanced at my watch, 2:30. We went south, then along First Avenue and up B Street. At B Street and Fourth Avenue you turned right to go home. I suggested going further up B Street but you protested, "We've been out almost an hour." "No," I said, "We left at 2:30, it's not been quite half an hour." You retorted: "At F Street I looked [at the time] and it was 2:13." You got angrier and angrier, saying that I lied and that you needed to "give me a lesson" on telling time. I said that you might consider the possibility that you misread the time [on your phone]. "No!", you said. Defensively you remarked, "Oh, I'm a dumb ass and can't read the time." You then walked away from me. You were angry and so was I. You said you will do what you do and that's that. TBI.

March 15.

Dear Adam:

After your mom and I got home from church I fixed you a Reuben sandwich. You came upstairs to eat. I mentioned that the Jazz lost in triple overtime last night. You said, "No, double overtime, I looked it up." I showed you the paper: (A1 section, upper right hand corner) "Three Ots the hard way. The Miami Heat outlasted the Jazz 140-129 in triple overtime, marking just the second triple-OT loss for Utah in franchise history. C7" Your response was, "No, the paper is wrong." Later, your mother and I discussed how rigid you are since your injury, how, like yesterday, you assert your views and are unable to accept the possibility of being incorrect, of having misread something. "Traumatic brain injury," she said. "I'm just grateful for what we've got."

It's now 2:45. I heard the door open and walked to the front window to look outside. You were about to cross the street, heading to church. You were not wearing a hat. A good sign, I think. You weren't trying to hide your scars.

March 16.

Dear Adam:

Today we left early for the University's Voice Disorders Clinic to meet with specialists on vocal cords and the damage caused by intubation. While waiting, you said, referring to the possibility of working with a voice therapist, "If this costs anything, I won't do it." Having others pay for your care really bothers you, an unwelcome sign of dependence. First you were checked out by Dan Houtz who had you do a number of verbal exercises, including reading (which proved difficult because of your vision—you had to hold the folder right in front of your face) as he listened and then looked at your vocal cords on a monitor while he made a video tape recording. After looking at part of the recording you commented, "If Kirby saw this she'd never kiss me again. Gross." It wasn't gross, but very interesting. You were embarrassed by some of what he had you do, for instance singing a little song and holding a note for as long as you could (16 seconds, it turned out; you noted you did 17 seconds in rehab). EEEE, low to high, high to low. PaPaPa... TaTaTa... PaKaTaPaKaTa...done as fast as you could (which wasn't very fast). The conclusion reached by Dan Houtz: "No lumps or bumps on the vocal cords, so this is good." There is some "maladaptive tension in the cords—squeezing front to back." Perhaps the most interesting moment came when Dr. Marshall said, after reviewing your case, that in a year or two you'll probably be fine. To which you said, "We've been given [such time frames before] but no one really knows." He agreed. So, talking and singing and, as always, patience. Therapy was not suggested.

> *Memory (age 4, July): "You sang almost constantly while we were in Ohio. The best part is that you are perfecting your vibrato! I love it when you wake up singing as you so often do and I love it even more when you begin a more or less familiar tune and, not knowing the words, create lyrics as you go acting as though they are obviously as good or better than the originals."*

> *Memory (age 12, December): "You were chosen to sing a number with a small group of boys at the school concert. You were very pleased. The teacher announced his selection in a wonderful way. You sang the song, then he turned to the boy who would be announcing the number at the concert and said, 'Say all the names of the other kids and put in Adam.' The class applauded."*

March 18.

Dear Adam:

At 11:30 you and I went for a walk to Memory Grove park. You were very somber, going only because I insisted that we walk. On the way you talked very little, commenting to just about everything I said or asked in these words, "I don't care" or "It doesn't matter." You said that at times you wish you were dead, that this is the worst time of your life—a statement you reiterated when I mentioned the story reported in the *New York Times* about an actress named Natasha Richardson, daughter of Vanessa Redgrave and wife of Liam Neeson, who has a serious head injury following a skiing accident. You said, "She's going to have the worst time of her life." You now seem resigned, that there is "nothing anyone can do" to help you. Seth came by after we got home and hopefully a little time with him will pick you up a bit. He's been a blessing. I heard someone downstairs playing the drums while you were strumming some chords, it was Seth. Later I said to you, "I didn't know Seth played the drums." "He doesn't," you said, it was his first time trying.

I love you. Dad

March 20. Day 220.

Dear Adam:

Sadly, Natasha Richardson died yesterday from her head injury.

It is 3:28 p.m. You are with your friend Alex, a drummer.

It's no wonder you get frustrated: you are dependent on your mother and me in ways you hate, even when you want to go get something to eat you must get someone to take you. Frustrating. Intimacy... Well, you and Kirby talk a lot during the day. If you are talking on the phone and either your mother or I come into your room (we knock), you stop talking and often get irritated by our intrusion. You get upset when you are writing on Facebook and I'm standing nearby even though I do not read what you have written. It's true, you have little privacy, and this interferes with your effort to establish intimacy with Kirby or your friends. Identity. I think a lot about this, of how your identity has been shaken by your injury—to a degree and at this moment you have lost much of your music, all of your athleticism, and many of your friends, and friends are an important part of who we are or who we take ourselves to be.

You are always very happy following a day spent with my parents. Yesterday you won the card games you played and were thrilled with the dry fly Dad painted on your drum cover, black on white. It really is neat. Dad was pleased to do this for you.

And More Bills

March 21.

Dear Adam:

Matt asked my permission today to ask Rachel to marry him. More changes!

March 24. Day 224.

Dear Adam:

Before leaving work today I phoned you to say I'd be home in about 50 minutes and that I'd stop by Subway to pick us up lunch. Concerned that you wouldn't like what I ordered, I wanted to know what you wanted on your sandwich; you suggested we go together. I got home about 2 p.m. We walked to Subway to get something to eat.

Once home we ate in the dining room where you had placed the sandwiches, talked, and then played four games of cards (Rachel said you and she played cards this morning. "He totally whooped me," she said). While we were playing the last game, Kirby phoned. You asked if it would be all right for you to call back later, that you were "playing cards with [your] dad." I liked how you said this—that what we were doing mattered to you. We had a very pleasant couple of hours together. I didn't nag. You didn't feel hassled. We need more moments like these.

March 27.

Dear Adam:

This afternoon you, Rachel, and I were playing a card game—good for your hands. The mail came which included a number of bills which really upset me. All along the way we have not been well informed. I should have studied our insurance policy, but when things were crazy I simply couldn't face it. Lots of confusion. For example, I didn't know that every year we start over on our deductible, the result of which is some bills came that I hadn't expected. When we were first told by Billie (who has been wonderful) not to worry, that we needed to focus on you and getting you well, I must admit I gladly let things go. Even with Yvette helping, I've missed a lot. Today, seeing bills from Gentiva, Rehab Without Walls, that included the phrase, "Collection Notice," on the top really threw me off. I phoned Yvette and was told we owe them, and, she said, the Trauma Group's bills have not been cleared, that there is nothing more to be done—so we owe these also.

I decided I should write to one of the Trauma Group physicians, which I did, to see if there is a possibility of an adjustment. Here's the letter:

Dear Dr. Caritas:

I'm writing on behalf of our son, Adam Bullough, who you may recall was admitted to Mission Hospital on August 12th following a fall on his bicycle.

First, thank you for the care you gave to Adam. He is doing well—very well, we are told, compared to what was expected. Double vision persists as do balance problems and weakness on his left side—no fun for a musician! We are working with a number of therapists and despite his struggles remain positive and hopeful. Since returning home he's had an additional surgery to remove the blood clot filter which went well.

Since coming home on November 14th, we've been trying to sort out the bills, mountains of them. Our insurance company, Deseret Mutual in Salt Lake City, contracted with Health One [of California] so payments could be made. We were never asked about coverage and were never told that any of the providers would not accept Health One. Only much later, when the bills started flowing, did we discover that the Trauma Group was not a contracted provider—had we known, of course, we would have insisted on some other arrangement being made with the hospital. The accountant who works with us at Deseret Mutual and with whom I meet about every other week—we talk more often—reports that twice efforts have been made to work with insurance groups that the Trauma Group will accept. I cannot claim to understand how all this works, one of the mysteries, but a month ago we were told that the second attempt was successful, not to worry. We even received several notices of payment from Deseret Mutual, indicating the account was mostly paid in full. I was lulled into a momentary peace. On March 3rd Galiana (who you know handles the accounts for the Trauma Group) phoned to report that nothing had been worked out, that Deseret Mutual was wrong in the assumptions made and that we needed to pay the billed amount. We are anxious to do what is right.

I don't know what options, if any, are available, but I thought I should write to you to see if anything can be done. We have bills from [several physicians in your clinic] totaling $5,898.48.

I must say, the events of the past several months have given me insight into the challenges of our medical system. If there is something that can be done, we'd be most grateful.

Thanks much.

Nothing may happen, and we may be stuck, but I thought this worth doing. I'm not certain Dr. Caritas even knows what has been going on. On the upside of the financial news, I made the last payment to Coast Radiology and I received a statement from the hospital saying that the bill has been paid in full. That's great news!

March 28. Day 228.

Dear Adam:

I spoke with an attorney, a family friend, this afternoon who deals with hospitals and insurance companies all the time. We were advised to write a letter to the Trauma Group telling them that they've gotten all they are going to get, that we are "done." "Legally," he said, "we don't have to pay for anything, the bills are [yours]." I don't feel badly about having paid some of these, but it does bother me we never had any say in the services performed by the Group. He said they should write everything off beyond what the insurance pays, that this is what is done. But we do feel responsible. If we have any difficulty he's offered to write a letter as our legal counsel.

Not Just an Injury

Dear Adam:

On Friday we begin the additional session at the balance clinic, now two a week. Soon we should have the name of the hand specialist Amy mentioned and we'll see where that goes. Your mother and I continue to be concerned because you are not pushing yourself even as we understand something about the intensity of your inner battle, a war between a weakened hope and despair.

I wish you could more fully understand how we love you, Adam. Your mother and I are trying to keep our focus on your well-being and not fall into discouragement ourselves, discouragement not because we believe you are not going to heal but because we see you sometimes working against yourself.

April 4.

Dear Adam:

Last night your mother, Aunt Tammy, Uncle Dan, Phyllis, Grandpa and I attended the Family Recognition Ceremony for organ donors to honor Grandma Mortensen. An amazing evening. Among other things a slide presentation was made that ran for 18 minutes showing the faces of people who are dead but whose organs were donated. (Grandma Mortensen would have been included but Grandpa missed the deadline to submit a picture.) Most of the 100 plus people were young men, about your age. As the music played and the slides changed, I glanced at your mother who was in tears. Both of us thought of you, and felt grateful we didn't need to make the decision that so many of those also watching had had to make. We are grateful for your life, Adam, so very grateful. Among the slides were three, as I recall, of babies, two days old or less, and a few little children. Lots of heartache but also lots of goodness.

Last night you attended your missionary reunion. Adam, whose last name I forget, took you. You said you were glad to have gone but you only knew a few people there. This morning as I tried to get you to share what had transpired you said something that really touched me. Everyone, you said, knew about your accident and then you made reference to your accident being the only thing that seems to matter, that everything that goes on is tied to it. As I thought about your comments, I realized how difficult this must be for you, that you have come to be defined by your injury and this is not who you are, or at least is but a small part of who you are or want to be. I think of Lisa Foto who has written so often on Caringbridge. She has done so very much for and been so very kind to those, like us, who have passed through Mission Hospital and struggled with TBI—but in doing so the danger is that the experience of injury can become wholly self-defining. I have got to do more to talk about and focus on other aspects of your life and being. I'm sorry.

April 5, Sunday, 7:30 a.m.

Dear Adam:

Mom and I began a fast yesterday, Saturday afternoon. A bit after 10 p.m. last night something very special happened. I was at the computer in the Study unwinding when suddenly I heard music. Quickly I shut down the machine and went into the bedroom where I found your mother standing, near you, while you were sitting on the bed strumming a Robert Johnson song. You wanted her to hear it. As I came in you kept playing. I watched and listened. You said you couldn't play the song all the way to the end, but you were sufficiently satisfied with what you could do that when I asked you to play it again you did. A week from today will be eight months since the accident, eight months. Your left hand remains disobedient, as you said, but it's healing and, for once, you admitted just a bit of optimism. We asked you about the troubling D chord, which you played, saying that sometimes your hand won't do it, but it did last night.

April 6.

Dear Adam:

This morning, early, we left for your appointment with Dr. Katz, a neuro-ophthalmologist at the University. You were really hoping for a simple solution to your double vision: glasses. Your eyes were tested and a resident, Dr. Wong, checked your body—reflexes, strength, touch as well as your eyes. After a wait, Dr. Katz came in and a discussion took place between Drs. Wong and Katz while a young woman stood by and listened. Later your eyes were dilated. The nerve to your right eye that pulls it to the right is not conducting properly; the brain and the body are not quite working together. Glasses really are not the solution, but you are a good candidate for surgery. You were, to say the least, very disappointed especially after being told that you'd have to wait another three or so months to make certain that your sight has stabilized. You understood me when I said that we "need to do whatever is best for the long term," but the words rang hollow. We'll meet May 12th with a surgeon who will, I think, establish a baseline against which to make additional measurements and this means more waiting. Before meeting with Dr. Wong you were quite hopeful, even talking about driving again soon. Your hopes were dashed, and we had a very tense drive home. We were both upset.

Three hours at the Moran Eye Center then at 1 p.m. you had a session with Amy in the Balance Master with the little green man. I received a phone call from Jeanette, the hand specialist, who will begin working with you on May 1st. She's looking forward to it. She has a copy of your cd and said she planned to listen to it soon. A good sign.

April 7.

Dear Adam:

It's 8:16 p.m. You are downstairs watching a DVD, "Big Trouble in Little China." You worked again today doing filing at Joshua's office for a couple of hours—for the experience, not pay—and this morning took Layla for a walk to the dog park in Memory Grove. Just before we were to leave for Joshua's office you said that you needed to stop by the bank "to make a deposit." You received your second tax return and wanted to deposit it so that you can buy presents for Kirby and others in California. This is typically you, generous even when you have little.

This afternoon I received another phone call from Galiana of the Trauma Group, first complaining about Deseret Mutual Insurance, saying that she had never dealt with an insurance company that is such a problem, that the company continues to try to find ways for reducing the bill. What a comment! I'm just grateful for what they have done and are doing. She said that she feels badly for us, that we are "caught in the middle." She said that the Group isn't going to accept the insurance as full payment, that they had received the letter I sent and that they would give us a "discount" if we paid the amount in full. If we opted for payments, we'd be charged the full amount. In response, I told her that I had spoken with an attorney and that he said we shouldn't pay anything, that "we aren't responsible." I said that you have nothing, and the prospects of you returning to work any time soon are dim. She turned icy cold. "Yes, you aren't leeegully responsible. I'll turn the account over to a collection agency." "Wait a minute," I said, "I'd like to talk this over with my wife. How much of a discount are you talking about?" "Thirty percent." I phoned Yvette at Deseret Mutual but she wasn't available. We spoke later. Some days ago she told me that Deseret Mutual planned to pay some more on the account, and I asked her what had happened. She did some checking, and reported back that there were still three bills being processed. The amount left for us to pay is "$3,139.79." So, if the bill stays at this amount, we'd owe, which is to say, you'd owe the

Trauma Group $2,197.85." The bill, dated February 4th, was "Past Due" and $6,919.87. Crazy. I cannot help but wonder what would have happened had we had no insurance whatsoever. Many of the patients in the Surgical ICU were in this boat. Near the entrance way of Mission Hospital is a posted statement that we passed day after day after day saying that no one will be refused treatment even if they cannot pay!

When your mother got home from work I told her what had transpired and asked what she wanted to do. She concluded that we need to pay the bill; she doesn't want you to have a bad credit rating, wants to be able to visit the hospital next week without feeling obligated, and wants to do what is right. To us this isn't a legal but a moral issue. So we'll pay and be glad for the reduction. We certainly do not want to take any chance that difficulties for you will arise from this situation at some future point. So, that's the story.

It's now 9:00 p.m. You came into the bedroom and announced, "I'm hungry." When you are hungry you simply must eat; waiting is not an option. You want a pizza, which we'll have tomorrow. Nothing else will do. As I write you are foraging in the pantry and are pretty irritated, speaking in Spanish under your breadth—this is a bit like what Nick Charles does in the movie, After the Thin Man, when waiting at the door to go into "Aunt Katherine's" house for an unpleasant New Year's Eve gathering. Standing by his side Nora asks what he is doing as he mutters. "Getting all the bad words out."

Memory (almost 2 years-old, February): "[Adam] you are an incredibly sweet and loving child. An example: today I gave you a couple of graham crackers. The first thing you did was march off toward the bedroom where Seth was watching one of his favorite violent cartoons, shouting, 'Seth, Seth, want a cookie?' When you got into the room you handed both of the crackers to Seth who, of course, gladly took them. Had I not told Seth that one of them was for you, you would have been left out in the cold, cookie-less."

Ties

April 16. Day 247.

Dear Adam:

You are in California and visited Mission Hospital with Mom yesterday. She wrote an update on Caringbridge while at the hospital. Daniel, Christine, and many of those who cared for you were there. Happily, no one was in room 16. I am so glad for this. It was a delightful reunion, your mother said.

I miss you. I really miss you.

Our neighbor Lia baked you another cake. She didn't know you were away in California and I didn't have the heart to tell her. I was riding the recumbent bike when the doorbell rang. I went downstairs, opened the door, and there she stood holding an umbrella and occasionally coughing as it rained hard. She said she had baked the cake but wasn't able to carry it and the umbrella at the same time. This was about 6 p.m. After finishing exercising I walked over to her apartment, as promised. She, Jared and I chatted as I held the cake in one hand, an umbrella in the other—and it got heavier and heavier. Lia has embraced you and our family and for this we are very grateful.

I don't get much done during the day. Mostly I wander around. Last night before going to a play I started a pot of stew. Today I need to clean out the frig which is full of rotting food. I read—been reading Charles Freeman's book, *The Greek Achievement* (a great book)—and try to make myself interested in university work. So, the funk continues. I've noticed memory lapses—I couldn't recall the name of Peracles' or Prometheus this morning, this despite running Peracles' name through my head yesterday.

April 23.

Dear Adam:

It is 6:47 p.m. Thursday. I was just out back in the next door neighbor's yard with you trying to find a "Cream medallion" that went missing you thought while you were playing soccer with your cousin, Lydia, and her friend Dax and a boy I didn't know. Dad picked you up today about 12:30 and took you to their place. I'm so grateful for your grandparents' help and support. You enjoy your time there. Shortly after arriving Dad said he didn't feel well, and went to bed. You and my mother had lunch together and then played pool—you won the last game when she scratched on the Eight ball. While playing pool you phoned me, mentioned that Dad was resting, and asked if I could pick you up earlier than planned, which I did. When I arrived I went into Dad and Mom's bedroom, where Dad was sleeping. Seeing him in bed in the day time was disturbing, a sight I actually do not recall before. Later, he came into the kitchen where Mom, you and I were sitting and talking. I mentioned to them that Joshua and Vorn are moving to Pittsburgh for Joshua to study to become an archivist. They want their grandchildren close by and the thought of Joshua and Vorn leaving was a little disturbing.

Yesterday I took you to the balance clinic for therapy. Amy had you jumping side to side and back and forth across the broad blue lines that run down the hallway. When you saw me, you told me to leave; you didn't want me to watch. Later, I snuck another peek, until you caught me again. You were walking heel to toe and having a very difficult time of it. After perhaps going about 4 feet you'd tip and steady yourself by placing your hand against the wall. We still cannot get you fully to understand the importance of working hard on these and the other exercises you've been given. You think that you'll just get well—or not—as the brain heals, seeing no connection—or not believing there is a connection—between physical activity and healing. We're told this is normal, however.

After the session was completed Amy asked if we planned to continue with the therapy. I was surprised by her question since I thought this had been decided before you left for California. I said we did, and she said that you will need to have a session with Dr. Ballard to set new goals, "that you had met all of the goals that had been set." News to me.

April 26, Sunday. Day 256.

Dear Adam:

It is 10:28 p.m. I just came upstairs after hearing you sing your new song. It's beautiful, and profound. I cannot adequately express my feelings watching you sing and play your guitar and harmonica (when you performed the song for your mother last night you used the base drum). I watched your face and left hand intently. How grateful I am for the blessing of your life and for seeing you gain back a measure of your musical skill. You are working hard to get your left hand to behave. Not easy. Your voice is different, a bit muffled, but as your mother said last night, it's getting better. And it is.

Keep Pushing, Keep Pushing

April 30.

Dear Adam:

Yesterday your therapy with Amy was cancelled because she was ill. The person who phoned mentioned that you need to be reassessed because they are thinking of "releasing" you. This was a surprising statement since I'd spoken with Amy before and told her we wanted to continue your therapy. I said that having a therapist involved was really helpful, a way of encouraging you to do therapy, for one thing, but also it's a way of informing you of helpful activities to do. She phoned back and tomorrow, Friday, you will meet with Dr. Ballard at 9 a.m. Afterwards you have your first appointment with the hand specialist, Jeanette. I'm so hoping what she is going to do will prove helpful.

Tuesday night a bit before midnight you weren't home. No one knew where you were and you didn't answer the phone. Although your mother's and my day had begun at 4 a.m., we were both worried and I was awake, in the Study, waiting and wondering. Finally, about midnight you answered your phone. You'd been at some sort of musical performance with a friend. I know, I shouldn't worry but I do. I drive you crazy, sometimes treating you as much younger than you are. Forgive me this insanity.

April 30.

Dear Adam:

Tonight we were talking and you said that you are always angry.

May 1.

Dear Adam:

We got home a little while ago from your therapy sessions with Dr. Ballard and with Jeanette Koski, a faculty member at the University, who specializes in brain injury and hand rehab. You are her first clinical patient; perhaps others will follow.

The session with Dr. Ballard began with him asking you about your exercises. You exaggerated what you do. Then, he reviewed your recent test results. I noted that the balance test last Friday reported that you once again scored a 78 composite, the same score you received two weeks ago. He said that was true, but that the printout showed that you were more stable, less wobbly, and that's good. So, while the scores are pretty much the same the computer showed there was less moving around as you centered yourself on the little green guy. He underscored that you are doing very well, and stressed the importance of working at the limits of your ability, that it is important for you to be challenging yourself. I mentioned that the range open for improvement has shrunk, which makes improvement of the composite score increasingly difficult. He agreed. He also tested your time getting up and running around a cone placed in the hallway. This score has continued to improve, starting at 8.9, then 5.3, and now 4.8 seconds. And, he had you working on a rocker board with your eyes closed, something that is very, very difficult for you to do without falling. Among other things, you are to keep working on the "tandem gait", walking heel to toe.

Jeanette is a delight. She's relatively new to the University and in addition to teaching occupational therapy classes also does all field placements. She did an assessment and the two of you began making plans for future sessions. She wants you to bring to the sessions activities that you value, part of encouraging you to work, I think. As the session began she admitted that she had anticipated you'd be in worse shape than you are, and she immediately rethought her plans. You liked her, a lot, saying that after I left

(I excused myself about 15 minutes before the session ended so I could book additional sessions with Amy) she warmed up more and "even told jokes."

You made a very interesting remark while speaking with Jeanette. You mentioned that you've noticed that drumming has helped you gain movement in your wrists, that when you started you used only your arms and shoulders. This surprised me. She said that when regaining mobility what happens is that gross motor functions return first and gradually, with practice, refinements follow—arms to wrists to hands and fingers. On the way home I asked why you hadn't mentioned this before. You said, "I only noticed it two days ago." Changes and being aware of changes are two very different things, and often help is required to notice improvements. Thus, the data Dr. Ballard reviewed with you.

Both Jim and Jeanette commented on how important it is for you to keep pushing yourself, that sometimes it is easy to give up, to decide that good enough is good enough. They said that you will likely need to keep doing your exercises—forever, I wondered?—else you will slip backward.

Monday, May 4. Day 265.

Dear Adam:

On the way to the Children's Museum to check on the possibility of a job you said that you wish you'd died, that dying would not be "as bad as this." Comments like these are heartbreaking. Generally you refuse to do your therapy when it involves activities different from what you used to do before your accident. We cannot get you to understand that you are not quite the same person you were before, and that given how conditions have changed, how you have changed, your actions also need to change. Hearing this, you clam up.

On the way home you again spoke about getting a Clapton guitar, saying that you need it because it has such a wonderful sound and that you need lots more instruments. Lack of money and wanting the guitar is the main reason you want a job. Until your sight improves there really isn't much you can do and, more to the point, you are not looking toward the future in any meaningful sense although, ironically, you speak about becoming a physical therapist.

New Opportunities

May 6, Wednesday.

Dear Adam:

I cannot help but think of your comment of a couple of days ago, that you wish you had died, that anything would be "easier than this." Not so, Adam, not so. How grateful we are for your life.

While I was in Provo at work yesterday you and I chatted briefly. You had just spoken with Julie Miller, your mother's principal, and agreed to return to teach PE at Wasatch Elementary until the end of the school year. Your mother told me that you told her that you wouldn't "be able to run with the children any more," but that didn't matter to her. You'll be at the school on Monday and Wednesdays, all day, which will be exhausting. Oh, but what a wonderful blessing this is. You seemed very pleased. We'll have to do some juggling of your therapy, but this is only a minor inconvenience.

It's now 3:30 p.m. Not long ago I returned home from your therapy session with Amy. I dropped you off at the Salt Lake City School District offices. (From the District you'll walk downtown to meet with folks at the Children's Museum—you said that walking would do you good since you have a long walk coming up next week for the Brain Injury Association of Utah and your legs are weak.) Amy had you work on the Balance Master, and took a couple of photos of you on the machine with Dr. Ballard standing nearby for the center's web page. After the photos were taken you worked on level 2 and 3 and did well. You have not worked at level 3 before. Then, she had you doing a kind of dance where you stepped on a pad on the floor that indicated on a computer screen whether or not you achieved the desired steps which were demonstrated by little characters. I wondered how you could see what was going on given your double vision.

The most important outcome of the day followed after you completed your session. We walked toward Amy's office where she would make copies of the results of your Balance Master performance for me. She asked you if you were riding the recumbent bike, which you admitted to doing only occasionally. Then, she asked if you were going to the gym with your mother and sister. You said that you hadn't, that they went at times when you "couldn't go." Not true. I mentioned to Amy that you refused to go, that you "hate gyms" (and I can't blame you). As you stood outside of Amy's (and also Dr. Ballard's) office, I followed her as she made the copies and told her you simply wouldn't go to the gym. She lowered her voice and asked if you might consider coming to the clinic to do a workout while she works with other clients. Perhaps, she wondered, you might want to do some volunteer work afterwards with Parkinson's patients. I thought this sounded wonderful. Returning to you, she asked: "Did Dr. Ballard mention to you the possibility of exercising here and then volunteering to work with the Parkinson's patients?" "No," you said. Then she explained what she had in mind, that often she needs help on Tuesdays and Thursdays from 10 to 3, a time when physical therapy students have courses and cannot assist her. She described some of the very accomplished people she works with, how interesting they are, and said that what you would be doing is talking with and encouraging them. It would, she said, be a very good experience "if you are serious about [becoming a physical therapist]." You seemed very pleased with the idea and said you'd really like to do it. So, this coming Friday she'll set up an exercise program for you which you will do before assisting her, I assume starting next Tuesday. Terrific!

May 16, Sunday, about 1:30 p.m.

Dear Adam:

Last night Kirby flew to Salt Lake for a visit. We bought her an airline ticket as part of your birthday present. Today we participated in the Brain Injury Association of Utah sponsored walk and then went to breakfast. I have to say, I delighted watching you jump across the finish line! While sitting in the restaurant, a fellow, noticing the Association shirts we were wearing, approached us and asked, "Who had the brain injury?" You spoke up, "It's me." He asked you how it happened and you explained, briefly, "an injury" riding a bike. He said that he was going riding shortly. Sometimes you wear your injury as a sort of badge of honor, something that gives you a special insight into suffering and a kind of moral cachet as one who has suffered. You're right, no doubt. You like the scars, and you are not shy in talking about your experience. I think this is healthy even as you desperately want to be normal.

The session with Jeanette on Friday really encouraged you. I hadn't imagined this, but there really are dramatic differences between therapy for hands when the focus is orthopedic compared to when the concern is the brain. Somehow I had imagined you spending endless hours picking up nuts and small bolts, but not so. She is working on your brain and your hands. (One of the activities she has you working on is building a bird feeder; sanding with your left hand is one of the activities she has you doing.) After your first session with Jeanette I realized it was best for me not to attend, that I make you a bit self-conscious. You've commented on how funny she is and how much you enjoy working with her. I'm thrilled. As instructed, you brought your guitar with you. She is a musician and has you work on specific skills. For example, you mentioned that there is a particular song that has a difficult riff that you used to play with ease. Since your injury it's very challenging. You are supposed to play these notes 20 times a day in four sets of five. She explained to you that by about the fifth time your performance would deteriorate, but that is normal, don't worry. When this happens she said you should stop then do a set a bit later, spreading sets across the day. She told you that it is her opinion that your hands will return to very near normal, words that really encouraged and lifted you. Apparently she bases this conclusion not only on how far you have come in the past few months but from her assessment of how your hand "feels." Like you, I was thrilled by what she said.

> Medical memo: "For decades the presumption was that the neuronal pathways and synaptic connections established during the brain's initial development were immutable. Today we know that the brain is capable throughout our lifetimes of adaptively modifying and

reorganizing the connective pathways that it has laid down, and that the development and consolidation of these pathways depends in quite a major way on how we use our brain and what for."

"[The] brain takes on the form of how it is used. The neuronal connections that we activate especially often and successfully in dealing with the world become more and more strongly developed, and the ones that are employed only quite rarely either stay the way they are or gradually begin to deteriorate. Since there are no two people who have had exactly the same experiences in their lives and have used their brains in exactly the same way, every brain—given the course of its particular history—is unique." [15]

Reconnecting

May 22. Day 283.

Dear Adam:

Yesterday you had your 9 a.m. session with Amy followed by a couple of hours working with Parkinson's patients. Afterwards you phoned me to report that Amy told the person who does the billing that there wouldn't be a charge for your session. This pleased you, I think, because you are earning your way. I mentioned that this frees up some money and perhaps we could fly Kirby in for the weekend. Last night, before prayer, you, your mother and I were chatting. I asked if you'd told your mother what had transpired. You said you had and got a big grin on your face and said that because of the therapy not costing anything I had mentioned the possibility of flying Kirby out. Then, you asked, slyly, "If she can't come could the money saved be put toward a Clapton guitar?"

Amy seems to think that you don't need her help anymore, that if you will do what you are supposed to do at home and meet with her on Tuesdays you'll be fine. Fridays you will continue your therapy with Jeanette. So, some good news.

I got home late last night—a long day. You'd cleaned up a lot, cutting back your beard and mustache. You looked great, not just less scruffy but positively handsome, I thought. This morning while we walked to the car to drive to Wasatch Elementary School I looked at the side of your head. From your scaring the hair is a little funny, but no one would really notice. You look good. I dropped you off on the corner by the school and waited as you walked across the street lunch and maté container in hand. Your gait isn't quite normal and you seem rather fragile to me but I couldn't help but think of how far you have come.

Yesterday Steve, who schedules for Dr. Dries, the eye surgeon, phoned. He couldn't get you an appointment for surgery until July 14th. I was disappointed and I know you are as well. Despite this, you said that he had done the best he could to get you in and that he'll try to arrange an earlier date if he can and will call in the next couple of days. This morning you again mentioned that we needed to listen to you earlier and not pay so much attention to the physicians, that if this had happened you would already be able to see better. You said this but there wasn't the sort of bitter edge that so often has accompanied your expressions of frustration. Perhaps this is a sign of resignation but I think not. Rather, I believe you are gaining greater control over your emotions and have a better understanding of not only your situation but of others'.

May 22 (second entry).

Dear Adam:

I just got off the phone with Gentiva, Rehab Without Walls. I thought we only had one more bill to pay with them but it turns out there are three. Still, we're getting closer to having these paid off. I'll be so very glad. Last night on the way home from work and picking you up at my parent's home you talked, as you often do, about needing to find work in order to purchase a Clapton Guitar. You insist that the instruments you have now are not good enough for what you need. I so hope you are right, even as I wish this obsession would pass.

You only have perhaps three or four more days at Wasatch Elementary teaching P.E. which heightens your concern for work. By the way, you've really been brilliant with the children. Last night I mentioned that we'll soon start working on the front porch and I'll pay you for helping. You said you also plan to call the Children's Museum again. I have to paint the dormers and re-roof the back of the house, but these are tasks you cannot do. You said, you "can't climb on the roof." I'm delighted that you are cautious, not pressing to drive or ride your bike before your really are able to do so without worry.

Rachel took you to your therapy session this morning, rescheduled because of Memorial Day weekend. Interesting. Jeanette brought a key board to have you work with certain chords. The point isn't to learn to play the piano, as you said, but to fire the brain and work the hand. You made a point of telling me that if you are to practice on our piano it has to be tuned, otherwise you are "not going to do it." Okay. Okay.

May 23.

Dear Adam:

It is 7:41 a.m. This morning Kirby flies in to Salt Lake.

Today I heard you play Sunshine of Your Love on your electric guitar. I cannot help but contrast what I heard with what I used to hear—you struggled as you played, there was little fluidity, and soon there was silence. I cannot imagine how you must feel.

May 30.

Dear Adam:

The session with Jeanette went very well. I spoke with her briefly before the session began. She said that she feels the two of you are "well matched" and that you are on the right track. You leave these sessions energized and positive. As we left the clinic you said that you had finished the bird feeder, that it wasn't very good and that had you had the "proper tools" it would have been better. Of course, it isn't the product that matters but the process.

Seth came by last night for a few minutes. So much of our attention right now is focused on you and also on Rachel. Joshua and Vorn have each other. Seth is the person left out. (I say this knowing that loneliness is an issue you also face.) As I fiddled with the computer he commented that if someone calls about his attending his high school reunion, don't answer, don't respond. He's worried about finances having just received a $1,000 bill for his last kidney stone. Fortunately, he had insurance else the situation would have been worse.

May 31.

Dear Adam:

Getting home I looked at today's newspaper. A1 had a long article on Peggie Battin, the wife of Brooke Hopkins, an emeritus professor of English at the University of Utah I knew. On November 14th, the day you got home from Mission Hospital, after teaching a class on Mark Twain for a group of "older" students he went on a bike ride in City Creek Canyon. Coming down the canyon he ran into another cyclist whose bike was destroyed but he wasn't hurt. Brooke got a broken neck and is paralyzed from the neck down. The article focuses on how, since the accident, Battin, a philosopher specializing in medical ethics, has had to face the limitations of her previous view of things. She no longer is able to maintain the distance she once had to the dilemmas that demanded her attention and focused her critical capacities. I mentioned this story to you, again underscoring what we discussed the other day about the Multiple Sclerosis and Parkinson's patients at the balance clinic: They can only expect to get worse; you can work for and get better. How blessed we are, even when it doesn't feel like it—I guess this is part of maintaining hope, of discovering seemingly for the first time that others really are worse off than are we. As we sat at the table playing cards you mentioned that Lisa Foto emailed you through Facebook, mentioning that room 16, your room at Mission Hospital SICU, is now occupied by a mother of three young children, the youngest only three months old.

June 2.

Dear Adam:

Today is your last day at Wasatch Elementary School teaching P.E. Being able to return to the school to teach has been a huge blessing for you and, I would add, for the children. Yesterday, Monday, was yearbook day. When I picked you up you were very happy, laughing you told me that you had a long line of kids waiting for you to sign their yearbooks. You mother made a similar comment. You said when you started signing the yearbooks you wrote something personal, looked up and saw a line of waiting children 50 yards long (given you see double, two lines 50 yards long...a daunting sight!), and then changed your plans and began writing, "Have a great summer. I'll see you next year! Adam."

Today you were supposed to do your volunteer work with the Parkinson's patients but because of the school schedule will need to reschedule to Thursday. Your alarm didn't go off this morning, so we didn't get to the school until about 8:40. I have to admit I enjoyed watching you scurry about getting ready, not wanting to be late. Yesterday you were the first one there, arriving at the school early to get everything set up for the children.

June 3. Day 295.

Dear Adam:

This morning I took you to the Children's Museum where you dropped off a note including a listing of the things you believe you cannot do. Your hope is that Martha will still hire you since, you said, they badly need help. You remain fixated on getting a "Clapton guitar" which you believe will help you to get back to your former abilities.

On the way home you talked about messages you'd received on Facebook. I asked if you had read Caringbridge recently. No, you said, not in about a month. I mentioned that your mother hadn't written in quite some time.

You responded by saying, "I should write on it." I encouraged you to do so even though it's probably the case that many folks have gotten out of the habit of checking the journal.

June 4.

Dear Adam:

You wrote on Caringbridge last night for the first time. Here is what you wrote, which is terrific!:

"Dear family and friends,

It's me, Adam. I wanted to take the opportunity to say 'hello' and thank all those who have supported me during this terrible time... Thank you all and I love you.

Things have really been getting better. I have started working again at the elementary school as a gym teacher and am loving every minute of it. The kids have been great and really seem to be interested in my progress. I don't go a day without hearing one of the kids say how glad they are that I am back. They speak for both of us; I am thrilled to be back as well.

On the 16th of May, Kirby came out to participate in the Utah brain trauma walk. [The walk] was so much fun. I really loved having her here with me and I loved to have my family go do that with me. I am surrounded with amazing people that make my life worthwhile despite the current conditions. My heart continues to belong to the guitar. Thankfully my ability to play is returning and I have begun to write music again.... I have a few new songs that I am quite proud of. I hope one day you will all get to hear them. I am so grateful for all of you and the support I receive from you all. I hope that everything is going well for you all and look forward to hearing from you. Thank you and I love you. Adam"

"Fun" Therapy

Dear Adam:

Yesterday you did some checking on eBay for a Clapton guitar. A 2004 model was offered for bidding starting at $1,699—the auction ends tomorrow early afternoon. Just imaging getting such a guitar gets you very excited. While you were still looking, in the kitchen your mother and I talked and decided, given how important this is to you, that we would try to buy it for you with the understanding that you would work to pay for it. I made the bid, the first. You were thrilled. Early this morning you went to the computer to check the auction and called out to me, "Dad, someone else has bid." You went downstairs and I got up and looked at the bid, thought about it for a few moments, and raised our maximum bid to $2,000. Our competition, as you discovered later, must be a dealer of some sort, having purchased more than 20 guitars over the past 30 days, usually with only one bid. His bid was the prescribed $25 more than ours. So, now we wait.

Fortunately, there is another Clapton guitar for sale, not necessarily for bidding—a "buy now" offering—so we have a backup plan: If we don't win the auction—We'll immediately purchase the second guitar which is a bit more. About 20 minutes ago, 7:20 p.m., you received a text message from Ashley Evans from Idaho asking about the auction. I asked you who it was. "Ashley Evans." "From Idaho?" "Yes." "You've told people about the auction?" "This is big for me, I'm so excited."

Tonight Rachel returns from her trip to California. A late flight to maximize the time she and Matt have together. Briefly I spoke with her earlier today about her arrival time. She was very happy.

As I write you and your mother are sitting on the porch finishing supper and talking. It's been a quiet day starting with us going to the hardware store to get a bolt to fix the pedal on your drum set and you visiting Corina Ayala to talk and drink maté. Mostly you spent the day alone, like so many days. Fortunately, tomorrow you do your exercise regimen and work with the Parkinson's patients at the balance clinic. (I am so grateful for Amy making this suggestion.) After school Lydia and Corina's daughter, Tootie, checked in, which you and they enjoy else they wouldn't visit.

June 9.

Dear Adam:

This morning I got up and looked to see how the bidding on the Clapton guitar was going only to find that we had been outbid. Yesterday you asked me to increase our maximum bid to $2,100, and I did. So, I called to you and we discussed what to do. There were still nearly six hours remaining before the auction closed but we decided, given who the opposition was, to simply purchase the other guitar. I had a heck of a time getting PayPal to respond, but finally it did and in a few days you'll have your guitar. It cost $2,199 plus shipping but we didn't want to risk you not getting one of the guitars even though this one did not have a pickup. This said, from the pictures, I believe it is in the better shape of the two guitars, showing much less neck wear indicating it has been played considerably less. I worried you would be disappointed, but you say you are not. (The deal is that you will pay us back and, more importantly to me, play for us!) Once this was done we went by the Museum where, once again, Martha was absent—I get the impression she is avoiding you. When I picked you up you said that the number two boss had been let go, which may be an indication of financial troubles.

At lunch we talked about this year. You spoke a bit about your struggles with discouragement, and I recalled the day in the hospital when you said, "Dad, I'm losing hope." That was one of the most difficult days of my life. We talked about the day that Seth flew to California and surprised you. I shall never forget the look on your face. Seeing Seth your eyes teared up and the two of you embraced. I am so grateful for Seth's kindness. He lifted you at a very difficult time, when the infection raged within you. We've come a very long way.

June 11.

Dear Adam:

In the morning yesterday you phoned to see if I'd been sent any information about when the Clapton guitar would arrive. I hadn't but shortly thereafter an email arrived, then another and another, giving this information. I phoned home but you were in the shower so I asked your mother to tell you that I had forwarded the emails to your address. The guitar is supposed to arrive on the 17th.

On the way to your rehab this morning you mentioned that Kirby and Heidi want to fly you to California for Kirby's birthday. You seemed very excited. Then you said that you'd like to stay for a couple of weeks. I'm not certain this is a good idea but no doubt you will do as you please. You are an adult.

June 12.

Dear Adam:

Ten months ago tonight you had your fall.

Today you had therapy with Jeanette. You always leave therapy happy. Seth and I took you, then Seth and I had a quick lunch and returned whereupon the two of you toured with Jeanette the body parts room of the anatomy lab at the University (near Jeanette's classroom). You were thrilled. I waited in the car. Seeing body parts in jars isn't something that I want to do. At lunch Seth and I spoke at length about his future. He wants to get on with his life—increasingly this seems to mean not doing hair. He said that he had never thought he'd cut hair for the long term, that he became a stylist because he didn't know what else to do. We also spoke about Zuriick, and his involvement designing clothing for the company. Seth reported that Zuriick is now making money, so....fingers crossed. As we drove home from therapy Seth pointed out four boys who were walking toward the 7-11 near the University on 13th South—three of them wore Zuriick shoes, perhaps ones like yours, shoes he designed.

June 16.

Dear Adam:

Tomorrow the Clapton guitar arrives. Boy, are you jazzed!

After spending the morning at the balance clinic where you did your exercises and then spent an hour or so working with people with Parkinson's disease (or a related disease) I made you lunch and then around 1 p.m. Lincoln came and took you to get some items you need for the guitar—new strings, a humidifier—which you said only uses distilled water (In earnest, you said, "and you ONLY use distilled water")—a tuner and something for Lydia. (It's fascinating how intensely you talk about some things, what needs to be done, in a way that has an urgency both in words and in affect—strong words, strong affect.)

At the clinic I had a long chat with Amy. She mentioned how difficult it is for people with Parkinson's, TBI and other maladies to stay engaged in rehab noting that they think they've worked hard for a long time but really have done very little therapy. By the way, Amy said that she's worked with other TBI patients and you are amazing. You'll be different than you were before the accident, she said, but what you have done and how far you have come given the extent of your injuries has really impressed her. Noting the plasticity of the brain, she stressed the importance of you working diligently, doing those activities that will fire the neurons forming the pathways that control your hands because, she said, if you don't you'll not gain in function.

On the way home we talked about your work with the Parkinson's patients, which you said you enjoy but it has been difficult, you said, to get to know adults: "I'd prefer working with children," you know and understand them.

One of the people you help at the clinic is Kurt, an Indonesian who studied in Germany with one of the physicists who guided the German rocket program during World War II—I thought it might be Heisenberg, but Amy didn't know. He's a "rocket scientist" who, you said, speaks five languages. Kurt comes to the clinic with his wife—he's bent over, to the side, and has real difficulty getting around. You seem really to enjoy your time with him. You also helped Hank, who is in a wheelchair and is, you said, the only person other than yourself who was there who doesn't have Parkinson's, although he has a related and more aggressive disease. "No one [with this disease] is supposed to live past their 20s and Hank is in his 40s." You thought he is being studied because he is so exceptional.

Tonight my parents are coming for dinner. Tomorrow will be an exciting day!

June 17, Wednesday.

Dear Adam:

A little after noon today the Clapton arrived. Being slightly unsteady, nervously and ever so carefully you carried the shipping box downstairs and anxiously opened it. It may be a day in June but the moment belonged to a Christmas in childhood. It is now a bit after 2 p.m. You are downstairs with Lydia, playing, having replaced the strings (which were new but not ones you like). You seem so happy. After your mother got home from the Temple together we went downstairs, and at our insistence you played for us. You chose to perform your new "situation" song. Before starting to play you had to tune the guitar, then clip a bit of excess from each string. Holding the guitar on your lap and a wire cutter in your right hand you used your left to hold the wires to cut. You had some difficulty getting hold of the strings to cut them, no doubt in part because of your double vision but also because of a lack of fine motor coordination. You had to retune the guitar but then played and sang. Your voice is slurred but you played well. We were thrilled.

I just walked downstairs and smelled spray paint. Nuts. I wish you wouldn't do this. I've asked you not to. The other day you made a stencil so you could put your name and a profile image of yourself on your various guitar cases. I guess this means the Clapton is home.

Gaining Perspective

June 21.

Dear Adam:

Today is Father's Day. As I write you, your mother, and her dear friend Diann are staying with Heidi and Kirby in California. I just spoke with you and your mother who reported that you and Kirby are getting along "great."

We returned a few minutes ago from my parent's house. I picked up all the makings for deli sandwiches and other stuff for lunch. My sister joined Vorn, Joshua, Seth, Rachel, Mom and Dad and me. We all sat around the table and talked as we ate. Lots of fun. It's especially wonderful to watch and listen to Rachel who seems very happy. For Father's Day in addition to lunch we gave Dad a family picture within which, because you were away, you had been Photoshopped in—you look about 6 foot 4 in one of the pictures—the fellow who did the insertion of your photo doesn't know you so perhaps he thinks you're a very tall guy when you aren't. It's funny, not only are you tall in the pictures (we gave Dad four of them so he could pick which one he wants to put in the frame we gave him) you face right and left—the image in some of the shots is reversed. Oh well.

Yesterday brought a surprise: Seth phoned to ask me to dinner. Sadly, I'd just eaten. He said that he was watching a documentary about a boy and his father, and that boy seldom expresses gratitude and often dismisses and mistreats the father. He said that he thought of me and wanted to express his appreciation. Laughing, he said that it just so happened that these feelings came the day before Father's Day. He's funny.

June 25, Thursday.

Dear Adam:

Today Michael Jackson died. He was 50 years old. Strange. I've often wondered what would become of him. Perhaps like me he couldn't imagine himself as an old man. His was a tragic life.

You and your mother are still in California.

At Lisa Foto's request today you and your mother visited with Jake, a twenty-six year-old young man, and his parents at Mission Hospital. Your mother said this is the first time you've actually seen anyone in the PSCU who was coming out of induced coma and it was an "eye opener." Perhaps now you will realize how far you have come in your recovery. Apparently, like you, Jake came to California for a girl but the situation wasn't working out. Your mother wasn't clear quite what happened to him but it sounds like he may have fallen. He's an alcoholic, and there is some thought he had been drinking. Like you he had a craniectomy but mercifully he did not get ARDS. He's been in the hospital since May 9th. For four or five days his parents, who live in the midwest, didn't know where he was so they filed a missing persons report. He was a "John Doe." Your mother said that visiting him seemed to comfort the parents who have been with him twice since his admission and have to fly home on Tuesday. She said you were encouraging to Jake, telling him to "Hang in there, it is worth it." The visit was a very good experience for both of you.

June 27.

Dear Adam:

It's 7:20 p.m. About 20 minutes ago I received a phone call from a young woman who said that she was our dear friend Charles Eads' niece, that my name was in his directory, and that he died last Thursday apparently of pneumonia. I shall miss Charles—his whistling, singing, kindness and smile. He visited here about three weeks ago. "How is your boy?", he boomed, thrilled to see you.

Our house is filled with reminders of Charles' generosity—from the mirror in our bathroom, to Rachel's bed, to the Victorian dresser downstairs in the guest bedroom to the round oak table I have yet to restore sitting in the shed. These are but few of the items we have that Charles found. Friendship like that offered by Charles to me is a rare and wonderful gift.

July 4, Saturday.

Dear Adam:

As I write you and Rachel are again in California. Rachel left Thursday; you left yesterday. She returns late tomorrow while you return on the 12th, I believe, the day before we meet with the surgical prep team for your eye surgery. Speaking of surgery: I spoke with Billie at DMBA about the possibility of plastic surgery to fix some of the damage on the side of your head. They'll pay for a consultation which will determine what can be done and, depending on what is found, will provide the basis for determining what, if anything, the insurance will pay for. Now, the quest for a plastic surgeon begins.

Thursday morning I took you to your appointment with Jeanette. On the way home you talked about your session. You said that the feeling in your left arm is changing, that it feels, as you said, a bit like what happens when a limb is starting to "not be asleep." You were concerned and asked her if this was normal and whether or not it is a good sign. You wondered if this was a sign that you have improved as much as you are going to improve. She reassured you, telling you that you will continue to improve, that you have not hit a plateau. I'm so very grateful for her, her knowledge, insight, and understanding of you. As I've said, you always leave these sessions happy.

(Dad commented that when he picks you up at the balance clinic you are very involved, working right in the "midst" of everyone. He commented on how "personable you are" and also mentioned that you told him that you hoped to do this sort of work in the future "but with children.")

July 8.

Dear Adam:

Yesterday you visited with your new friend at Mission Hospital again and wrote a really wonderful CaringBridge entry. Well done, Adam, well done! Mom and I are grateful you have reached out to Jake and can see how he, in turn, has positively influenced you, helping you better to understand your own journey. As you note in your update, he understands the lyrics of your recent songs as no one who hasn't trod a similar path as yours could. You also mentioned that because he so enjoyed your music you feel encouraged to play for others.

Seeing Straight

Dear Adam:

Today is Kirby's birthday. Tomorrow you return home. Monday is the appointment with Dr. Dries to check things for Tuesday's surgery.

Yesterday was the one-year anniversary of Grandma Mortensen's death. At 2:15 several family members gathered at the grave site in the Provo City Cemetery. I actually left the office about noon and went to the grave site to have some quiet time with Grandma. I miss her.

We gathered at 2:15, went to a restaurant for a late lunch or early dinner— we waited forever there to get our food and ended up being late for our 5:20 tour of the Oquirrh Temple which was recently completed. Vorn, your mother and Seth rode with me, and Seth was really on one—he was so very funny. At one point we were talking about names that Vorn likes for a child. I guess Seth has learned to say a few Hmong phrases, and he went off on what it would be like to name a child Pa (soft a... Paaaa), said with the proper tone. How could anyone ever be angry with someone named Pa? He was incredibly funny. Good to laugh. I haven't done much laughing lately.

July 12.

Eleven months since your accident, Adam.

I picked you up at the airport this morning from your stay in California.

With me I brought the Clapton guitar, sitting in the back seat. I told you that he insisted on coming to the airport with me and wouldn't take "no" for an answer, that he got pissed off when I tried to dissuade him, so, here he is. You smiled.

When your mother and I got home from our meetings you were downstairs working on a song, Clapton in hand.

I'm glad you are home, Adam. Love, Dad.

July 14.

Dear Adam:

It's 9:15 a.m. Eye surgery at 12:30. Your mother and I have been fasting. Last night my parents dropped by to wish you luck. They worry.

10:25 p.m: Here's today's report: We got to the hospital about 12:15, you filled out some more forms, and we waited. About 2:30 you finally were taken in for surgery. About 3:45, Dr. Dries came and spoke with us reporting, with a smile, that the surgery went beautifully, and saying that he was very "optimistic" about the long-term results. Once he began surgery Dr. Dries decided that the muscles on both eyes needed adjusting. Shortly thereafter your mother and I went into the recovery room to be with you. You were groggy, and funny. Your eyes were very bloodshot. You were given intravenous anesthesia which allows for greater control, so your recovery was very fast. When we told you that Dr. Dries said the surgery went beautifully you said, "That's because I'm beautiful." Later you couldn't remember having made this remark nor, I should mention, recall speaking with Kirby on the phone. You wanted to talk with her. By the way, in the recovery room you peed twice, once with a bottle, a skill that you perfected at Mission Hospital. So, lots of good news.

Tomorrow at 10:45 we have an appointment with Dr. Dries who will check to make certain your eyes are aligned as they should be. Despite being quite uncomfortable, you seem very pleased with the result. You see double if you keep your head still and look sharply up and to the sides. Dr. Dries said this was likely, but you don't seem to be bothered by it. You are taking pain medication, as needed, and for the next 14 days will have eye drops to prevent infection and swelling. The sutures will dissolve on their own. What Dr. Dries did was weaken the medial rectus muscles on both eyes to compensate for the lateral rectus muscles so both sets of muscles can work better together, more in balance.

That is the report.

"Life is like that"

July 15.

Dear Adam:

You were up all night, unable to sleep. You spoke with Kirby until 3 a.m. and were wound up thinking about all that is going on in your life. When I walked out of the bedroom this morning you had placed the white board you used in Mission Hospital for writing near our door propped up on a cushion so that the following message was easily and unavoidably read: "Mom & or Dad, Please make sure I get up and moving on time, I don't know what time my appointment is. Adam." Actually, you got yourself up and we were at Primary Children's Hospital to meet with Dr. Dries in plenty of time. Your eyes are very bloodshot, sensitive and sore, but working together as they should. You've noticed a sluggishness in how your eyes focus and move but, as Dr. Dries said, supporting what I told you when you mentioned the problem this morning, that this is to be expected having just had surgery. With time, this should improve. Dr. Dries was very pleased with the results of your surgery. I couldn't help but quip, "You are very pleased with yourself." And he was. No adjustment in the sutures is required. The sutures, by the way, are tied like shoe laces, one in each eye, and will dissolve over time disappearing in about two months. Despite your discomfort, already you have commented on how much easier it is to read. So, yet another good day.

We have an appointment with a plastic surgeon for August 5th.

July 16. Day 338.

Dear Adam:

You had a wonderful day today with my parents and Aunt Patio. I am so grateful for them and their ongoing interest in you. As we left their home Dad gave me three baskets of delicious raspberries he and Patio picked, some of which we ate on the way home. At dinner tonight we had raspberries and vanilla ice cream.

July 19.

Dear Adam:

It is now 7:10 p.m. Matt has been here since Friday. His plane leaves in a couple of hours. We had a very nice dinner together that your mother planned. We talked quite a while. I hope he comes to feel comfortable with our family even as I imagine it can't be easy. Joshua was pretty intense, as he often is. He's worried about their move to Pittsburgh and his return to graduate school. He'll do well. You seem to like Matt, which is important. I don't envy him taking the bar at the end of the month but I admire how he has focused his energy and how goal directed he is. At one point you commented that he and Rachel owe you big time since it was because of your accident they met. We laughed as we talked about you moving in with them as payment for your troubles, Matt suggesting that they build a pool house just for you. It's a good plan.

July 21, Tuesday, 11:13 p.m.

Dear Adam:

I just went downstairs to check on you and, seeing you, sat down on the couch. I asked if you are nervous about playing the Clapton at Mission Hospital on the 12th of August, the one year anniversary of your accident. You said that you are, that your "voice sucks" and that your hand won't do what it is supposed to do. I wanted to explain to you that those who will hear you perform that day will be people impressed with what you can do, and not concerned with what you cannot do. They know how far you have traveled over the past year. Still, you struggle and worry that you'll never be able to perform again at a high level. I mentioned to you what Jeanette said, that she expects your hand to return to full functionality in time, but my words fell flat. I'm so glad she has videotaped you playing. Seeing these tapes will help you recognize how you are improving.

Today you mentioned that you've shifted the keys of each of your songs downward, from E to D to accommodate the change in your voice and that you need a new harmonica, a D, so you can play "Going to California", one of your "best songs," you said. To pay for a pickup for the Clapton guitar you traded your electric guitar, not the Ibanez, for credit. You worry about money but until your eyes heal getting work will be difficult. Part of me wanted to pay for these items, but I've decided it is best not to, part of encouraging you to take charge of your life.

July 23, Thursday, Day 345.

Dear Adam:

It's 12:43. In a few minutes I'll be taking Vorn and your mother to the airport for their flight to Pittsburgh to find a place for Vorn and Joshua to live. No doubt they'll have a busy but wonderful time together. Vorn refers to your mother as "Mom" and me as "Dad," and does so comfortably. She's quite amazing and, I think, very good for Joshua.

Early this morning I primed the north and east dormers while your mom rode the recumbent bike. I'll ride later today. I hoped to beat the heat, and so started painting about 6:30 a.m. Finishing up, and a bit shakey—heights really bother me and now I'm a bit unstable—I showered, rested a little, and then took you to the balance clinic. You took your guitar with you and actually played part of the time while the Parkinson's patients exercised and after doing your own exercises. You said that you did this not primarily for the patients but for yourself, saying that you wanted to practice playing before a group of people in anticipation of playing at Mission Hospital next month. On the way home I asked you how it went: "Better than I thought it would." You said your voice was "okay." One of the reasons you were excited about going to the balance clinic today was that you hoped to speak with Dr. Ballard to see if he could fill out whatever forms are required for you to again drive a car. Jim wasn't there. You were told he had cancer surgery. We didn't know he was ill. On the way home you and I spoke about Jim's situation, how he has been working to help you and others overcome their problems while he has been struggling with his own. "Life is like that," you said. And it is.

This morning I spent some time reading materials on the book of Job preparing for Sunday's lesson. The story certainly captures many aspects of the struggle to come to terms with the problem of evil, of how bad things happen to good people. Three of Job's "friends" press him to admit that his life fell apart because of some sin even though Job denies it and his friends don't have any idea of what sin he possibly could have committed. A fourth friend, Elhu, a younger man, chastises the three, arguing that sometimes we suffer to protect us against greater sins, to warn us, and to increase our love for, trust of, and dependence upon God. Of course, not one of the four says that bad things happen because, as you said, "Life is like that." Crap happens. Tonight Jim will be in my prayers.

Nagging

July 27. Day 349.

Dear Adam:

Friday was the 24th of July, the Pioneer Day celebration. Your mother and Vorn were in Pittsburgh seeking housing and getting to know the area. Last night Joshua and I picked them up at the airport, late. They had a wonderful experience, loving the city and Stanley, the fellow who manages the building where the apartment Vorn rented is located.

Today you have three tasks awaiting you, and I've been nagging you about one of them: You've got to get your student identification number so you can again get enrolled in the community college. Given the lousy economy, enrollments are way up and I worry you won't be able to get into the classes you need. The other two, you're working on: 1) finding someone who can give official approval so you can drive again; and 2) finding a helmet so you can once again ride a bike, a helmet, as I said, that covers all your important parts—one that goes below your butt! (I like the image—two skinny, fury, legs poking out of a large, round, ball of brightly colored plastic with a visor! If this doesn't work, then bubble wrap and duct tape will do.) Nothing less will do! You made an appointment with Dr. Ryser to get approval to drive but it's more than a month away and you really do not want to wait.

July 29.

Dear Adam:

The past few days I've been nagging you, something you hate almost as much as I do. I've been trying and trying to get you to get your student number so you can register for fall classes at the community college, but, for whatever reasons, you wouldn't. It turns out that they wouldn't give you your number over the phone so you had to go get it. Then, with the number in hand you went on-line to register only to discover you didn't have the list of courses you needed to take given you by your counselor in May. Another trip to the college followed, this time with Rachel. Happily, when you got home you enrolled in two courses, psychology and communication. You might have thought this would end my nagging, but, alas, not so: I began nagging to get you to check on your application for financial aid. What followed was unbelievable: You phoned and were told that there was yet another form that you had not filled out, a form, you said, that you'd never seen before. I believe you. After all the time we've spent filling out forms this year we should be more skilled than we are.

July 30, Friday.

Dear Adam:

As I write you are with my parents. Despite your protest yesterday you got up early so we could go to the community college so you could fill out the missing aid form. From there we went to the balance clinic. At noon Grandpa Bullough picked you up for the day.

It is still Friday but now 5:27 p.m. I just returned from downstairs where you were lying on your bed. I asked if you knew where your mother is, you said "No." We talked briefly. Earlier today you got the Clapton back but without the electric pick-up installed that you need for the Mission Hospital performance. You were sent the wrong pick-up. The guy who is doing the installation is going to get another which will be installed on Tuesday, August 4th. We leave for California on the 7th. I said that you seemed "down." "Why wouldn't I be?," you said. With the Clapton in hand earlier you played and recorded some music then listened to the recording. You said you are not "half," not even a "fourth" as good as you were, and you "hate it." Of course I said what I always say, you'll never get back all your ability if you stop playing. You commented that it has been a year since the accident and you thought you'd be much further along in your rehab by now. This has been an enduring concern. Again, you spoke of how you sometimes wish you had died and that you'd be better off. I said, "I wouldn't have been." "You guys would have been fine," you said. Not so. Not so. So, the battle continues. Clearly, you are very worried about performing at the hospital on the 12th.

A Last Surgery

Dear Adam:

It's 3:38 p.m. As I write you are downstairs playing the Clapton and singing one of your new songs.

August 3.

Dear Adam:

Today you had an appointment with Dr. Dries at 2:30. Before the appointment his assistant checked your eyes and you gave her a copy of the form you need filled out so that you can once again drive in the hope that he can sign off. Not just any physician is allowed to sign these forms and we are uncertain he has the authority. Just in case, you have an appointment with Dr. Ryser in September for this purpose but we're hopeful you will be able to cancel.

Seeing you, Dr. Dries smiled broadly. As a "student doctor" looked on, he began checking your eyes. "You are healing very nicely," Dr. Dries said. And you responded, grinning: "You guys didn't make me a cyclops. Next time!" Lots of laughter followed. Dr. Dries had you look at a wall chart with your head held at different angles, right, left, up, down. You see double only when you look to the extremes, up, to the right and left—not down. "How is your reading?" "Fine," you said. "You are an easy patient." "I think you'll have a nice outcome the rest of your life." Dr. Dries was extremely pleased with the results of the surgery, as are you. He then filled out the paperwork required for you to drive even asking if I thought you were able to drive. I said that recently we paid the insurance on your car, to which he said, "that's a strong endorsement." You have the form waiting to be mailed tomorrow. Hopefully, this will do the trick, otherwise we'll have to wait until the appointment with Dr. Ryser next month.

August 5.

Dear Adam:

Tonight Matt arrives, late, bringing with him his dog. So, Layla will meet her future playmate this evening. The specific reason for Matt coming is for he and Rachel to get their wedding pictures taken. She seems excited. Tomorrow evening she has arranged a potluck barbeque here so everyone can meet Matt who hasn't. I didn't know this was going on until I received an email announcement from Rachel. Funny. The wedding is scheduled for January 9th.

This morning we had an appointment with a plastic surgeon, Dr. B.C.K. Patel, who was recommended by Dr. Dries. On the way you gave Mom and me grief, saying that you wouldn't have anything done if it required cutting your hair. It's taken you a year to grow your hair out and cover your scars and you aren't about to allow anyone to mess with your locks. You say you don't care about how you look, but obviously you do. I urged you to think in the long term, that there might come a time when you will want to have shorter hair. You thought not, saying that if being a physical therapist meant cutting your hair then you didn't want to be a therapist, that the work is stupid. What could we possibly say to a comment like this? I urged you to be patient, to listen to Dr. Patel and hear what he has to say.

The meeting was fascinating. Dr. Patel speaks quickly, efficiently, and helpfully. He examined your head, talked about the options, which involve a "volume augmentation" to the right side where your head is sunken. When asked what he would do if the patient were his son, he said there is really nothing to lose, that the worst case scenario is that you will be as you are. You then popped your question, that you didn't want your hair cut. You were relieved to hear that this isn't a problem, that the procedure is minimally invasive. Using the CAT scan on file, he explained what he saw, a loss of tissue—the temporalis muscle. The skin is now on bone and you have a diminished blood supply in the area, a potential source of difficulty but one that can be managed he thought. He was confident that he can much improve how you look and that you will be pleased with the results. He also noted that he might be able to remove some of the plates in your head which can be felt—I showed you where one of the screws is which you thought was just a bit of skin or bone. He answered my insurance question, saying that he knows how to gain approval for the procedure, a concern raised when I spoke with Billie—it must be medically justified. He then took some pictures, spoke into a recorder for a record of the meeting, and took us to the office of the person who sets his appointments. Your surgery is now set for early October. I think each of us left the meeting very optimistic. Most importantly, you'll get to keep your hair!

Love, Dad.

August 6.

Dear Adam:

Late yesterday afternoon you and your mom picked up the Clapton, who is now home and getting a workout pickup in place.

Today, while I was in Provo, your mother took you to the balance clinic where you exercised and worked with the Parkinson's patients. You also spent some time with Corina. Tonight was Rachel's potluck, which, although the evening began late, starting at 7:30, turned out well. Matt's dog, a boxer, and Layla had some difficulties—they fought tonight at least three times. (I have my doubts that the two of them are going to get along.) Matt met more members of the family, and seemed comfortable. As the evening wound down two delightful events happened. Matt's birthday is the 20th of this month. We gathered in the dining room and sang "happy birthday" and your mother gave him his presents from us. He was delighted. Then, you played two songs on your guitar with my parents, Patio, and several other family members gathered around you in the sitting room. With some urging, Lydia, who just got a guitar for her birthday and who you have been teaching, began playing slowly, deliberately, the Cream song, "Sunshine of your love." On February 2nd you tried to play this tune but couldn't. Tonight, once she started playing, you joined in and played well, both feet tapping time, you smiling and encouraging Lydia and coaching her.

Tomorrow, we leave for California and your performance at the hospital. A long drive.

Reunion

August 11.

Dear Adam:

Today we visited SICU to check things out for tomorrow's performance. While there we visited briefly with a few of your nurses who were delighted to see you. Fun.

6:32 p.m. You were practicing your guitar and singing. "Adam," I said, "you sound good." "Not good enough."

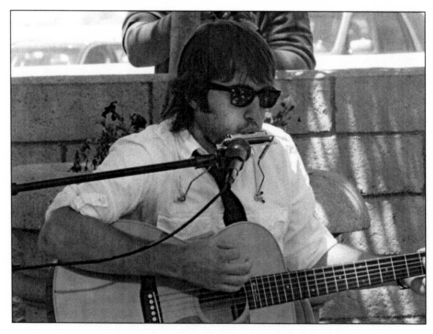

First anniversary performance at Mission Hospital

August 12. Day 365.

Dear Adam:

An amazing day! You wanted to get to the hospital early so we left about 10:15 a.m., stopping on the way from Heidi's house to purchase fruit and cookies. Others, it turns out, also kindly brought cookies including Sue Mordin. We had no idea how many people would come to the hospital to hear you perform and I suspect we all worried just a bit that few would attend. We arrived at the hospital about 10:50 to get situated and set up. Shortly thereafter Melinda Bahr, Jack, who is now four, and little Amanda, students in Heidi's preschool, arrived, happily greeted you and then sat nearby and ate lunch. A trickle of people followed as we got ready. Gradually the gathering grew and grew. Lisa Foto had phoned some folks and word spread even though it appears the flyers your mother sent to the hospital never arrived. Soon there were more than 60 people, including Michelle and Daniel who sat right in front of you, and other of your nurses, Lauri and Carol, some of your therapists, a couple of physicians and many other friends: Robert Ramirez and three other "survivors," as Lisa Foto described them, Dee Burrows, her daughter-in-law and grandson, the Mordins and many others. Susan brought Karen and her caregiver. As always, seeing Susan was a delight. She's a wild woman with a huge smile. It's hard to believe but today she surpassed herself. She is now the proud canvas for a new tattoo, her "brain tattoo," as she said, showing us. It's a brain, all right, purple with a red spot indicating the location of Karen's aneurysm, and includes Karen's name and "SICU" in bold letters.

Noon came. Then five minutes after. Everyone, and I mean everyone, was excited to see so many friends. Hugs. Lots of hugs. Pictures and more pictures—survivor pictures, family pictures—were taken. Lisa Foto then took charge. She introduced the survivors in attendance, five of them including herself, each still in one or another way recovering, introduced Diana Mordin who showed two survivor paintings she has completed, making a print for each survivor. I shall always be grateful to Diana for the lift she and her brother gave you when they decorated your hospital helmet with the stickers they designed for you—maté leaves and Clapton.

You then began to play and sing. Everyone, I think, was astonished by what they heard—I can only imagine what had been expected. As you sang your voice got stronger and, as Seth remarked, it was better than just the evening before. People came and went. When you finished, nearly an hour later, the hugging and talking resumed. Gil, another one of your nurses, commented on how seeing you and the others made his life meaningful. Your mother spoke with Mary Kay Bader, the force behind the SICU, who told her that the day before had been terrible, that she "had about had it" but today, she said, "I am filled and joyful." Later Mary Kay told me a story I hadn't heard before. She was in Cleveland when the call came asking permission to use nitric oxide on you, that she phoned a friend in St. Louis who "downloaded" his knowledge into her brain and she gave the go-ahead. She said that she has presented your case at Columbia Hospital in New York including playing your song, "Play for Me," and pictures of you. The story, she said, really touched those in attendance who asked, "Do you have these outcomes often?" "Yes," she said.

Some people lingered. Just before leaving the hospital I went into the SICU and stood in room 16, which mercifully was quiet, and thought of all the hours we spent with you there. I thought of the pictures of you, of friends and family, we taped on the walls surrounding your bed, of the sounds of the machines, and the beep of the monitors and the small indicator lights, green and red. All was silent. I walked past the Wall of Fame and all the posted survivor pictures, which now includes a new set of you your mother put together showing your progress over these several months. As I walked past the nurses' station I glanced toward room 14 with the large window where you first sat up and tried so hard to lift your head off your chest. At the other end of the hallway Michelle stood working at her computer just outside a patient's room. I walked toward her. She looked up, smiled, and said she had downloaded a picture of you playing that she had just taken. As you played I had noticed her tears. We hugged, I thanked her, and she said, glancing at your picture. "It's a miracle. We were ready to say 'goodbye' to him, and we never do that unless we are sure." She then smiled: "I said to [Adam], I wasted a lot of tears on you!"

We went to dinner and then took your mother to the airport to return to Salt Lake for her workshop on the 13th. Three times since we arrived in

California we have gone to the site of your accident hoping to deliver a box of chocolates and a card to the woman who helped you right after you fell by bringing towels for your head. This evening we tried again and still she wasn't home. On a long shot I knocked on one of her neighbor's front doors. Eventually a man answered, standing on the second floor outside balcony having just gotten out of the shower, he said that he was the one who called 911 and has wondered what happened to you. He told us his neighbor is a nurse working a night shift. You put our address on the envelope of the thank you note and we left the chocolates for her on the front porch.

We now know more precisely where you fell, and I think we have found the culprit, a raised, hard, plastic, street reflector embedded in the asphalt that certainly is large enough to turn a thin bicycle tire.

A wonderful day, Adam.

August 13, 2009.

Today we got up early to return home. I am so glad that Seth decided to come with us and not just because I needed help driving. For much of the trip the two of you sat in the front seats together talking, joking, laughing. Over the past few days he and I have also talked a lot, including about how the events of this year have affected us. We've each changed. Family is certainly more important than it was and some things just aren't very important any more. We've all grown, Seth said, and we are better people.

Arriving at home your new bicycle helmet had been delivered as well as a letter from the State of Utah, Department of Public Safety, Driver License Division. The first paragraph of the letter reads: "Based upon a thorough evaluation of your Functional Ability Evaluation and/or Certificate of Visual Examination, it has been determined that one or more driving restrictions are required on your driver license or driving privilege card." So, what is the restriction? "Corrective lenses." Only corrective lenses.

Love, Dad

September 11.

Dear Adam:

One last entry. I thought everything was in place for you to drive again, but no. Dr. Dries signature was rejected, only Dr. Ryser's would do. So, this morning at 11 a.m., you met with Dr. Ryser to get cleared to drive. In anticipation of driving again, you and Seth worked on Desmond. His battery was dead so before you left for your appointment you had it charging. We left about 10:30. On the way to the appointment you were very tense and blew up saying that your mother and I had promised you that we would take you driving this week but we didn't. You were very angry, complaining that no one pays attention to you and no one understands how difficult life is for you. "Damn head," you said, smacking yourself. I got very upset. I'd planned to take you driving and said, yesterday or the day before, that I'd take you before your appointment, and I meant it. I didn't realize how anxious you were, that you really weren't sure you would be able to drive. Somehow you had gotten the idea that you would be tested this morning, and you weren't certain you would pass a driving test. You also wondered, "What will I say if Dr. Ryser asked me if I am able to drive?" Arriving for your appointment about 20 minutes early I pulled the car into the large and almost entirely vacant west hospital parking lot, stopped the car—as you protested, angrily—got out, walked to the passenger side and told you to drive. Reluctantly, you got out, walked around the car, sat in and adjusted the driver's seat, and then drove, easily and well. You relaxed and I told you to drive toward the South building, where you had the appointment, and park. Which you did, lining the Edge up perfectly between the painted parking lines. "That answers that question," you said, obviously very relieved. During the meeting with Dr. Ryser you answered questions, were tested, and revealed that you had successfully driven. Dr. Ryser responded by saying that he didn't think you needed a driving test, that you seemed a "very low risk" for driving. So, no test. Dr. Ryser was delighted with how well you are doing, that you are back in school, as I told him, and even working—two items he thought very important for your recovery. The now properly signed form for the state to reissue your driving license will be—

probably already has been—faxed and soon you will be cleared for driving. This is an important step toward independence and toward regaining control over your life. I'm thrilled and no doubt so is Desmond.

Postscript

I have heard doctors say, 'If you don't have your abilities back by six months after your stroke, then you won't get them back!' Believe me, this is not true. I noticed significant improvement in my brain's ability to learn and function for eight full years post-stroke, at which point I decided my mind and body were totally recovered." (J. B. Taylor (2006). *My stroke of insight*. New York: Viking, p. 111)

During his appointment at the University of Utah's Voice Disorders Clinic on March 16th Adam was told that his voice would probably be fine in a year or two, that he didn't need therapy. Adam's response proved surprising: "We've been given [such time frames before]," he said, "but no one really knows." Reading the words quoted above, that following a stroke Jill Taylor noticed "significant improvement" for "eight full years" puts comments of this kind in perspective. As Adam said, "No one really knows." Jill Taylor has an advantage over most people struggling with brain injury: As a brain scientist she understands the nature of the changes that take place over time and has the ability to recognize improvements. Early in Adam's recovery, changes took place that were easily identified and progress seemed assured—one day he couldn't sit on his own without tipping over and a few days later he could sit on the edge of the bed for ten minutes and more; one day he couldn't lift his head off of his chin, a few days later he could; one day he couldn't stand, a few later he could take a few steps. Changes of these kinds, improvements in gross motor coordination, were dramatic. In contrast, especially given the nature of Adam's injuries, regaining fine motor skills comes more slowly, much more slowly. It was only on April 5th that Adam was able to make a D chord, and even then his left hand continued to be uncooperative. That Jeanette Koski, his hand therapist, videotaped him playing the Clapton proved crucially important for Adam to gain perspective—he could see that over time he was making progress, albeit very slowly. The scores of his performance in the Balance Master at the University's balance clinic served a similar function, offering proof of improvement, however slight. Like Jill Taylor, Adam has "desperately needed people to treat [him] as though [he] would recover completely" (ibid). But nothing is more convincing of improvement than data, hard data. Moreover, for some of us in Adam's life reviewing such data proved sustaining as we tried to convince Adam, and sometimes perhaps ourselves, that he would recover, completely.

Other sorts of changes are not so easily documented, changes in how he engages with and thinks about the world. As previously noted, early in rehab Adam thought he would be completely healed in a matter of weeks, certainly by May, a mere nine months after falling. It is now October. He is part way through his first semester back in school and doing well in his courses even though reading is more difficult than before. He understands everything. Again he is teaching P.E. at Wasatch Elementary School on Mondays and Wednesdays and is immensely enjoying the time he spends with the children. With the children he is in charge, engaged, more his old self. He is driving and becoming increasingly independent, but he is cautious when out and about when formerly he was fearless. So, part of Adam's former life has returned, more or less, but he and his life are both different. How he is different is a matter of occasional discussion. He says mostly he cannot tell how he has changed but he knows there are changes. Many issues that used to excite his imagination and boil his blood are no longer of interest. He had large numbers of friends and among them was often the one who planned and organized activities. He was very playful; others were drawn to him. Now, he spends more of his time quietly, often alone. His humor has not fully returned; and there is a serious and raggedly sharp edge to his personality formerly missing. He is often very blunt. He seems a bit emotionally flat, disengaged or, better said, preoccupied—but not when he is teaching P.E. He says he is less creative musically than before, that ideas do not come as easily nor as quickly as they used to but, happily, they still come. Multitasking is difficult. And he is easily angered, particularly when a course of action upon which he has embarked is interrupted. Discouragement often raises its ugly head. We have suggested counseling or a support group might be helpful where he would encounter people who are working on the challenges of TBI but for now Adam doubts the value. Looking ahead, there is good reason to believe improvements will follow. This is so in part because many of the changes we have noticed are very likely the result of having experienced and of living with the aftermath of a terrible injury and not of the injury itself.

Not all of the changes are negative, and these must be seen in the wider context of Adam's abundant abilities: he is still bilingual, musical, smart, and interesting. Gradually, he has become more concerned about his future. A few days ago, for example, while I was working in Provo he phoned and we chatted. He said he needed to go to the balance clinic to speak with Dr. Ballard, that he knows what he wants to do with his life: become a pediatric therapist who specializes in brain injuries. He wanted to talk with Jim about what is necessary to achieve this aim. As I thought about this conversation I realized that I had never heard Adam talk quite this way before. The tone was different. As we spoke, I mentioned that working with injuries of this kind means working with people whose "recovery doesn't go well," suggesting that the work is extraordinarily demanding and implicitly asking: Are you sure you are up to this? In response he mentioned what both Dr. Jensen and Dr. Chang have said, that the highs offset the lows. Further, he remarked that at one time he didn't think he could deal with challenges of this kind, but that now he knew he could, after all, he knows what's involved with TBI. One side benefit of this focus is that he is more determined to do well in school; and more so than any time since sixth grade, he is studying. A tutor is helping him get around some difficulties, getting and staying organized and with strategies for recalling information.

Adam has always been a generous person, but now there are signs of developing a deeper, more mature, sense of gratitude and of obligation. These qualities are expressed in numerous ways, most especially in a deepening desire to give back to those who have done so much to aid his recovery over the past several months and to help those who are suffering the consequences of injuries similar to his, people like Jake who he met on one of his return visits to Mission Hospital. I do not think he has ever felt such obligations before. In this respect, he is not alone: Each of us intimately involved in Adam's battle for life and subsequent recovery has developed a deeper understanding of how our lives are intertwined and of how interdependent and needy we all are, every one of us. This also is a positive outcome.

As I have written, TBI is not like other injuries nor illnesses. Over the past months Adam has had to develop a kind of Sisyphean patience, of having to do over and over again what often seem pointless acts in the hope that they will prove therapeutic and help him heal. To continue healing, he must continue therapy; at some point he will have to do therapy not so much to get well but to avoid deteriorating, as the therapists have said. Patience must be joined by persistence and determination since there is no telling just how much of his former self he can reclaim. While severe brain injury inevitably forces a longing and backward gaze, driven by mourning for lost abilities and a lost self as well as a wish to be the person one once was, healing requires finding new channels for the expression of the self, new stories and new patterns of human engagement and activity. While Adam is more than a survivor, his and many other survivor stories contain the stuff out of which new and potentially hopeful and powerful selves can be born—tales of struggle and disappointment but also of courage, great goodness and generosity, and of small and large triumphs. Miracles do happen.

Yesterday, October 9th, Adam had yet another surgery, this one on the bone-flap side of his head, an augmentation. A few screws were removed and the largest of the plates was adjusted, flattened out at the edges. One of the benefits of this surgery is that Adam's head is now a bit wider and his glasses better stay put. We do not know whether or not additional surgeries will be needed. On November 8th a new addition to Mission Hospital will be dedicated with a new SICU. Room 16 will forever be gone; so will Room 17 disappear, where Bobby, Mr. Han, and Manny died—nothing familiar will remain. Adam has been asked to come and play his guitar and sing at the dedication, a celebration long in coming. That will be a wonderful day! At his next birthday Adam automatically will be removed from our health insurance policy so in the next few months somehow we must find a new insurer, one he and we can afford. Compared to where we have been, this is a small thing, not even a bump.

Afterword: Time, Perspectives, and Hope...

A trauma team targets the first 60 minutes after a traumatic brain injury as the "golden hour" when interventions are geared toward saving the life of the victim. A critical care team thinks in terms of hours. Interventions are geared toward minimizing the secondary impact of the injury thus maximizing the recovery potential. In contrast, families think in terms of minutes, hours, days, weeks, months, and even years. Families think of survival and of life. Above all, they hope! Hope is the fuel that sustains families of the TBI patient.

Collectively, the goal of the team of practitioners and family members of a TBI patient is to save the life of the patient. Pressed on what it means to save a life, most would qualify the goal and speak of the quality of that life. Simply, the life saved would have a meaningful existence; not merely exist. Since the critical brain injured patient presents in coma with brain bruises, bleeds, and swelling, the outcome of the team's efforts are often unknown. The TBI team works diligently from the minute to minute interventions in the Emergency Room, Operating Room, and the Intensive Care Unit (ICU) through the days and weeks it takes for the rehabilitation team of practitioners to strengthen, mobilize, and refine the skills a patient needs to function in everyday life.

The journey our TBI patients take during these times is long and arduous. For the hospital based TBI team, this journey is often filled with critical moments when the team faces the challenge of pulling the TBI patient through life and death situations. The physicians, nurses, and therapists labor intensely while the patient is in the hospital, sharply focused on recovery. Our perspective of the experience of injury, though, is markedly different from the experience of the patient and family. *Adam's Fall: Traumatic Brain Injury—The first 365 days* chronicles the thoughts, fears, frustrations, and hopes of a family living through one of the most harrowing experiences a parent, sibling, or friend may have. Reading this story opens this experience for medical practitioners who often see only the beginning and not the end. It serves as a reminder to practitioners who care for TBI patients and to the families of TBI victims that while our goal may be shared our perspectives are very different. Adam and his family's journey teaches us that our interactions and conversations often are understood very differently, and that it is important for medical practitioners to come to understand the family's perspective.

Physicians and nurses should keep in mind that the early interactions with families make powerful impressions and sometimes have lingering consequences. Here it is worth noting the evolution of the family's relationship with Dr. Chang, beginning with what was felt to be an impersonal encounter to the development of trust and friendship. As Adam said following a visit to California and dinner with Dr. Chang, they now are on a "hugging basis." To this day, Dr. Chang continues to play an important part in Adam's recovery. Nurses' interactions with families are the most frequent and intense. Nurses should be aware that families are able to "accurately identify" their personalities and practice habits. Mission's SICU nurses work diligently to create a culture of caring. As is clear from the story, valuing the part an encouraging family presence plays in healing, they welcome family members to the bedside, share information, and engage them in the care of their loved one. The long hours spent working together often lead to long-lasting relationships and friendships, and this too we see. For nurses, such experiences increase job satisfaction and offer both professional and personal rewards.

Reading *Adam's Fall* has affected how I think about my work. Before reading the book, I gauged the outcomes of our patients from visit to visit noting improvements in their neurologic states. I believed rehabilitation was difficult but knew little of the many challenges that patients and families endure during the months that follow returning home. As I read of the ongoing struggle of Adam's recovery and of his battle with depression and anger, I came to more fully appreciate the importance of the family in a TBI patient's journey toward health. Without the persistent effort to continue rehabilitation, Adam would not have achieved all that he has regained. Bob's belief that to stop rehabilitation would halt Adam's recovery is telling. The need to educate insurance companies on the value of continued rehab treatments is of paramount importance. Each of us must advocate for our patients' recovery; saving a life is only a first step! This translates to becoming activists in bringing a change to health care practices that impose arbitrary limitations on rehabilitation services and thereby limit the potential for improvement in quality of life.

The outcomes of individuals sustaining TBI fall along a spectrum from death to something we call a "good recovery." Even in the best medical centers, there will be some patients who do not survive injury no matter what is done or how diligently we work. For these patients and their families, our duty is to do our very best for them but once there is no hope for life our responsibility changes; we must help the family grieve and begin to heal. Survivors also need help—family and friends who advocate and work for their recovery.

In Adam's case, his family brought such love, faith, and hope for his recovery that I have come to believe that they equally share the credit for Adam's healing with the hospital's TBI team. The take away message from reading this book is...Never, Never, Ever Give Up Hope!

Mary Kay Bader, RN, MSN, CCNS, Neurology and Critical Care Clinical Nurse Specialist, Mission Hospital, Mission Viejo, California.

References

1. Jian, J., Xu, W., Wei-Ping, L., Gao, G., Bao, Y., Lian, Y. & Luo, Q. 2005) Effect of long-term mild hypothermia or short-term mild hypothermia on outcome of patients with severe traumatic brain injury, *Journal of Cerebral Blood Flow & Metabolism*, 26, pp. 773-74.

2. Bigatello, L.M., Stelfox, H.T. & Hess, D. (2005). Inhaled nitric oxide therapy in adults—opinions and evidence, *Intensive Care Medicine*, 31, p. 1014.

3. Griffiths, M.J.D. & Evans, T.W. (2005). Inhaled nitric oxide therapy in adults, *New England Journal of Medicine*, 353, p. 2693.

4. Slutsky, A.S. & Hudson, L.D. (2006) PEEP or No PEEP—Lung recruitment may be the solution. *New England Journal of Medicine*, 354:17, p. 1839.

5. Broccard, A.F. (2007). Prone position in ARDS, *Chest*, 123, pp. 1334, 1336.

6. Bayir, H., Clark, R.S.B., & Kochanek, P.M. (2003). Promising strategies to minimize secondary brain injury after head trauma. *Critical Care Medicine*, 31(1), p. S112.

7. Zurn, A.D. & Bandtlow, C.E. (2006). *Regeneration Failure in the CNS: Cellular and Molecular Mechanisms* in M. Bahr (Ed.), *Brain Repair*. New York: Springer, p. 55.

8. Deller, T., Haas. C.A., Freiman, T.M., Phinney, A., Jucker, M. & Frotscher, M. (2006). Lesion-induced Axonal Sprouting in the Central nervous System. In M. Bahr (Ed), *Brain Repair*. New York: Springer, p. 102.

9. National Institute of Neurological Disorders and Stroke, National Institutes of Health, Information page, p. 13.

10. Wikipedia

11. Stein, D.G. (2000). Brain injury and theories of recovery. In A. Christensen & B.P. Uzzell (Eds), *International handbook of neuropsychological rehabilitation.* New York: Springer, p. 29.

12. WebMD.

13. Crow, S.F. (2008) *The Behavioural and Emotional Complications of Traumatic Brain Injury.* New York: Taylor & Francis, p. 56.

14. Neirynck, J. (2009). *Your brain and your self: What you need to know.* Berlin: Springer, pp. 21, 29.

15. Huther, G. (2006). *The compassionate brain: How empathy creates intelligence.* Boston: Trumpter, pp. 13, 85-6.